Psychopharmacology and Child Psychiatry Review

Psychopharmacology and Child Psychiatry Review

With 1200 Board-Style Questions

Prakash K. Thomas, MD

Yann B. Poncin, MD

Child Study Center
Yale University School of Medicine
New Haven, CT

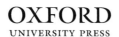

OXFORD
UNIVERSITY PRESS

Oxford University Press, Inc., publishes works that further
Oxford University's objective of excellence
in research, scholarship, and education.

Oxford New York

Auckland   Cape Town   Dar es Salaam   Hong Kong   Karachi
Kuala Lumpur   Madrid   Melbourne   Mexico City   Nairobi
New Delhi   Shanghai   Taipei   Toronto

With offices in
Argentina   Austria   Brazil   Chile   Czech Republic   France   Greece
Guatemala   Hungary   Italy   Japan   Poland   Portugal   Singapore
South Korea   Switzerland   Thailand   Turkey   Ukraine   Vietnam

Published by Oxford University Press, Inc.
198 Madison Avenue, New York, New York 10016
www.oup.com

Oxford is a registered trademark of Oxford University Press

ISBN-13: 978-0-19-974468-8

This material is not intended to be, and should not be considered, a substitute for medical or other professional advice.
Treatment for the conditions described in this material is highly dependent on the individual circumstances.
And, while this material is designed to offer accurate information with respect to the subject matter covered and to be
current as of the time it was written, research and knowledge about medical and health issues is constantly evolving and
dose schedules for medications are being revised continually, with new side effects recognized and accounted for regularly.
Readers must therefore always check the product information and clinical procedures with the most up-to-date published
product information and data sheets provided by the manufacturers and the most recent codes of conduct and safety regulation.
The publisher and the authors make no representations or warranties to readers, express or implied, as to the accuracy or
completeness of this material. Without limiting the foregoing, the publisher and the authors make no representations or
warranties as to the accuracy or efficacy of the drug dosages mentioned in the material. The authors and the publisher do
not accept, and expressly disclaim, any responsibility for any liability, loss or risk that may be claimed or incurred as a
consequence of the use and/or application of any of the contents of this material.

9 8 7 6 5 4 3 2 1

Printed in the United States of America

on acid-free paper

For our patients who share their lives and teach us.

Preface

If pediatric psychopharmacology adopted the same assessment, diagnostic, and treatment approach given to adults, then this book, as well as the text upon which it is based, would likely be an addendum to a general psychiatry text. On the contrary, the second edition of *Pediatric Psychopharmacology: Principles and Practice* speaks to the exponential complexity of assessing child and adolescent neuropsychiatric conditions. This comprehensive text of over 50 chapters by more than 100 authors provides an exhaustive update on the current knowledge of this field. In turn, *Psychopharmacology and Child Psychiatry Review* is intended to recapitulate the latter text in a question-and-answer format to help in retaining the many facts and facets of psychopharmacology and pediatric psychiatry.

Each of the six tests comprises 200 questions to mimic a boards-style format for the reader interested in preparing for the boards, recertification, or the child psychiatry resident-in-training examinations (PRITEs). We randomized questions obtained from all chapters of the parent text to represent the range and variety of psychopharmacology and child psychiatry in each of the six tests. In addition, the question stems and answers were kept brief and pithy—not just to imitate the style of boards exams, but to pare down the material to enhance the didactic point. We trust the reader to investigate the original text to obtain further details and citations.

In writing questions based on *Pediatric Psychopharmacology*, we kept in mind two primary goals: emphasizing material most likely beneficial for the study of boards, recertification, or the PRITEs, and including conceptual and historical material essential for a greater understanding of contemporary pediatric psychopharmacology and psychiatry. We do not believe it sufficient to supply a collection of facts on pharmacology, as that provides only a superficial snapshot of this rapidly advancing field. Consequently, we included questions that delineate the development of child psychiatry as well as areas of present uncertainty. At times, the questions and their explanations emphasize the provisional nature of our contemporary knowledge; yet familiarity with the forays into the uncharted domains of child psychopharmacology will help us to comprehend future advancements. In sum, we intend this review book of questions to engender even more questions in the reader, as well as an anticipation of what more may come from this emerging discipline.

We would like to thank Andrés Martin for the book's inception: he planted the idea of this review in our minds years ago. We thank the team from Oxford University Press who guided this publication to fruition, which includes Craig Panner,

David D'Addona, Kathryn Winder, and Molly Hildebrand. We thank the many authors of *Pediatric Psychopharmacology*, for it was a pleasure to read and translate their chapters into this review. And the continuing support of our families encouraged us toward the fulfillment of this work.

Prakash K. Thomas
Yann B. Poncin
Yale Child Study Center
New Haven, Connecticut

Contents

Psychopharmacology and Child Psychiatry Review

Test 1 Questions

1. **Which antipsychotic is likely to have the greatest risk for extrapyramidal symptoms?**

   A. Olanzapine

   B. Risperidone

   C. Quetiapine

   D. Aripiprazole

2. **Which group of youths in the United States has the highest psychotropic prescription rates, according to commercial datasets?**

   A. Uninsured status

   B. Low socioeconomic status

   C. Moderate socioeconomic status

   D. High socioeconomic status

3. **High rates of non-adherence to medication treatment (up to 50% or more) have been reported for a number of pediatric chronic conditions, including:**

   A. Asthma

   B. Epilepsy

   C. Diabetes

   D. All of the above

4. **Antidepressant drugs enhance neurogenesis in which area of the brain?**

   A. Hippocampus

   B. Thalamus

   C. Hypothalamus

   D. Prefrontal cortex

5. **Which is the correct order of length of clinical effect, from shortest to longest?**

   A. Dextroamphetamine, mixed amphetamine salts, methylphenidate, osmotic-release oral system methylphenidate

   B. Methylphenidate, dextroamphetamine, osmotic-release oral system methylphenidate, lisdexamfetamine

   C. Lisdexamfetamine, methylphenidate, dextroamphetamine, osmotic-release oral system

   D. Methylphenidate, lisdexamfetamine, extended-release mixed amphetamine salts, dextroamphetamine

6. **Which two medications have randomized controlled trials with reduction of aggression as the primary outcome variable, with results that have been replicated across at least two studies?**

   A. Methylphenidate and valproic acid

   B. Risperidone and valproic acid

   C. Lithium and risperidone

   D. Methylphenidate and risperidone

7. **Valproic acid has been used in the treatment of all the following conditions EXCEPT:**

   A. Epilepsy

   B. Bipolar disorder

   C. Migraine headaches

   D. Schizophrenia

   E. Panic disorder

8. Norepinephrine is released into the synapse from neuronal vesicles. Which drug(s) facilitate this release?

    A. Desipramine

    B. Amphetamine

    C. Methylphenidate

    D. B and C

    E. A and B

9. What fraction of the thirty to forty thousand protein-coding genes in the human genome is expressed in the central nervous system?

    A. One-twentieth

    B. One-tenth

    C. One-fifth

    D. One-third

    E. One-half

10. What percentage of youths with major depression report psychotic symptoms?

    A. 2% to 5%

    B. 5% to 10%

    C. 20% to 40%

    D. Over 75%

11. Maintenance treatment with medication is recommended for which of the following adult populations diagnosed with major depressive disorder?

    A. Those with three or more episodes

    B. Those with second episodes associated with psychosis

    C. Those with second episodes associated with prominent suicidality

    D. All of the above

12. The inhibition constant, K_i, is an indicator of:

    A. The effect of a drug

    B. The half-life of an inhibitor

    C. The method of metabolism

    D. The potency of an inhibitor

13. What is considered the gold standard in genetic linkage studies for the association between a genetic marker and a trait?

    A. Family-based studies using the transmission disequilibrium test (TDT)

    B. Randomized controlled trials

    C. Genome-wide scans

    D. The use of knockout mice

14. Which of the following describes the chief function of the cerebellum?

    A. The gateway for all incoming sensory information to cortical processing

    B. Temporal processing of motor and cognitive information

    C. The internal representation of sensory information

    D. Integration of input from cortical areas

15. Which agent was first developed with the intent to treat psychosis but was later marketed as an anxiolytic?

    A. Aripiprazole

    B. Chlorpromazine

    C. Olanzapine

    D. Buspirone

16. Which of the following statements is TRUE for children and adolescents?

    A. Most children and adolescents on Medicaid rolls are in foster care

    B. The greatest increase in rate of prescriptions is for antidepressants

    C. Males are more likely to receive psychotropics than females

    D. Blacks are more likely to receive psychotropics than whites

17. Tricyclic antidepressants were first developed as what type of agents in the 1940s?

    A. Hypnotic

    B. Antidepressant

    C. Anti-emetic

    D. Diuretic

18. **Which of the following therapies has the broadest evidence for anxiety disorders?**
    A. Individual cognitive behavioral therapy
    B. Psychodynamic psychotherapy
    C. Interpersonal psychotherapy
    D. Group cognitive behavioral therapy

19. **A "mixed" episode of bipolar disorder is defined by the DSM-IV as a discrete period during which:**
    A. Symptoms of mania predominate over depressive symptoms
    B. Symptoms of depression predominate over manic symptoms
    C. Symptoms of mania and depression are present but neither predominates
    D. None of the above

20. **Which of the following statements about neuroleptic malignant syndrome (NMS) in youths is accurate?**
    A. Second-generation antipsychotics seem to be associated with a more benign course of NMS
    B. A comparison of a case series of youths who developed NMS on first-generation antipsychotics with a case series of those who developed NMS on second-generation antipsychotics found that mortality was equal in both groups
    C. Bromocriptine appears to prolong the duration of symptoms
    D. NMS does not appear to occur in youths

21. **The temperamental attribute of behavioral inhibition may be a sign in childhood of increased risk for which condition?**
    A. Major depression
    B. Social phobia
    C. Generalized anxiety disorder
    D. Dysthymia

22. **Fluoxetine has FDA approval for what disorder or disorders in children and adolescents?**
    A. Generalized anxiety disorder (GAD)
    B. Posttraumatic stress disorder (PTSD)
    C. Obsessive-compulsive disorder (OCD)
    D. A & B
    E. B & C

23. **Kava-kava, an herbal preparation used to promote sleep, has been associated with which safety concern?**
    A. Eosinophilic myalgia syndrome
    B. Hepatotoxicity
    C. Acute renal failure
    D. Thrombocytopenia

24. **A meta-analysis study reported that the LEAST common symptom of mania in children and adolescents is which of the following?**
    A. Increased energy
    B. Distractibility
    C. Pressured speech
    D. Hypersexuality

25. **The primary intention during the continuation phase of treatment for major depressive disorder (MDD) is to consolidate remission and prevent relapses. For how long does this phase last?**
    A. 1 to 2 months
    B. 2 to 4 months
    C. 6 to 12 months
    D. 36 to 48 months

26. **Which of the following is most likely to lead to hypotension and bradycardia?**
    A. Venlafaxine extended-release
    B. Clonidine
    C. Norfluoxetine
    D. Amphetamine salts
    E. Guanfacine immediate-release

27. **What term describes the saturation of drug metabolism resulting in capacity-limited elimination?**
    A. Zero-order kinetics
    B. First-order kinetics
    C. Linear kinetics
    D. None of the above

28. The ability of rating scales to determine treatment effect is largely dependent on which two factors?

    A. Face validity and inter-rater reliability

    B. Construct validity and inter-rater reliability

    C. Criterion validity and inter-rater reliability

    D. Construct validity and respondent reading level

29. Which of the following best describes the effect of stimulants on blood pressure and heart rate, respectively?

    A. Increase in blood pressure of 3–4 mm and increase in heart rate 1–2 beats per minute

    B. Increase in blood pressure of 10–14 mm and increase in heart rate of 10–12 beats per minute

    C. Increase in blood pressure of 18–22 mm and increase of heart rate of 16–21 beats per minute

    D. Inverse relationship of blood pressure and heart rate, with increase/decrease in blood pressure of 3–4 mg and opposite decrease/increase in heart rate of 1–2 beats per minute

30. The antagonism of dopamine D2 receptors in which area of the brain leads to hyperprolactinemia?

    A. Mesocortical

    B. Nigrostriatal

    C. Mesolimbic

    D. Tuberoinfundibular

31. Total body water decreases rapidly from birth. At what age does total body water attain adult values?

    A. 1 year

    B. 3 years

    C. 6 years

    D. 12 years

32. Antipsychotic medications are prescribed most often in children and adolescents to treat:

    A. Psychotic symptoms

    B. Aggression

    C. Stereotypies

    D. Bizarre behaviors

33. What is the prevalence range of Tourette's disorder?

    A. 3 to 10 per 100

    B. 20 to 25 per 100

    C. 3 to 10 per 1000

    D. 40 to 70 per 1000

34. What percentage of pediatric patients receiving clozapine may discontinue because of neutropenia or agranulocytosis?

    A. 80%

    B. 50%

    C. 25%

    D. 5%

35. Which of the following is the mechanism of action of mirtazapine?

    A. Antagonism of presynaptic alpha-2 receptors

    B. Indirect increase of serotonin through adrenergic stimulation of raphe neurons

    C. Antagonism of 5-HT_{2a} and 5-HT_{2C} receptors

    D. All of the above

36. Which of the following pregnancy-related changes leads to overall reductions in lithium levels across pregnancy?

    A. Increase in total body water

    B. Increase in glomerular filtration rate

    C. Increase in transaminase metabolism

    D. A and B

37. Which agent has the longest half-life?

    A. Diphenhydramine

    B. Methylphenidate

    C. Hydroxyzine

    D. They all have approximately the same half-life

38. Studies aimed at examining the pharmacokinetics and toxicity of new treatments are called:

    A. Phase 0 trials

    B. Phase I trials

    C. Phase II trials

    D. Phase III trials

    E. Phase IV trials

39. Mild symptoms of tremor, incoordination, and confusion progressing to shivering, sweating, hyperreflexia, and agitation, and then to fever, myoclonus, and diarrhea are findings suggestive of which of the following?

    A. Stevens-Johnson syndrome (SJS)

    B. Neuroleptic malignant syndrome (NMS)

    C. Central serotonin syndrome (CSS)

    D. Malignant catatonia

40. Which statement accurately reflects clinical care of attention-deficit/hyperactivity disorder (ADHD) when a comorbid tic disorder is present?

    A. Stimulants should never be used

    B. The FDA suggests stimulants should be used after alpha agonists have failed

    C. Methylphenidate appears to be better tolerated than amphetamine

    D. There are no studies of stimulants for ADHD in tic disorders

41. Some researches have called obsessive-compulsive disorder (OCD) which of the following?

    A. Hyperglutamatergic syndrome

    B. Hyperserotonergic syndrome

    C. Hyperdopaminergic syndrome

    D. GABA deficit syndrome

    E. Hypercholinergic syndrome

42. Which of the following is considered the most effective agent for tics based on available data?

    A. Pimozide

    B. Fluphenazine

    C. Risperidone

    D. Clonidine

43. Which problem with memory is seen with benzodiazepines?

    A. Loss of memory for faces

    B. Anterograde amnesia

    C. Retrograde amnesia

    D. Loss of autobiographical memory

44. All of the following medications affect glutamatergic function in neuropsychiatric disorders EXCEPT:

    A. Lamotrigine

    B. Amantadine

    C. D-Cycloserine

    D. Gabapentin

    E. Memantine

45. Guanfacine immediate-release and extended-release have similar elimination plasma half-lives. What is the primary difference between these two formulations?

    A. The prolonged rate of dissolution of guanfacine extended-release

    B. The alpha-2 receptor selectivity is improved with guanfacine extended-release

    C. Guanfacine extended-release is eliminated by the liver, whereas the immediate-release form is eliminated by the kidneys

    D. Guanfacine extended-release is more potent

46. When abuse is suspected, what is a clinician's primary obligation?

    A. Talk to the parents as soon as possible

    B. Send the child to the emergency room for an evaluation

    C. Report it to child protection services

    D. Schedule a follow-up appointment

47. Zolpidem is metabolized through which two P450 enzymes?

    A. CYP7A1 and CYP7B1

    B. CYP1A2 and CYP2C19

    C. CYP3A4 and CYP2D6

    D. CYP39A1 and CYP46A1

48. Buspirone is an anxiolytic that acts as an agonist at which receptor?

    A. D_2

    B. $5\text{-}HT_2$

    C. $5\text{-}HT_{1A}$

    D. Alpha 2_A

49. Which of the following is one of the strongest predictors of a positive outcome in the treatment of adolescent substance use?

    A. Age of treatment

    B. Family involvement

    C. Group treatment

    D. The adolescent having a romantic partner

50. Which of the following is the only mood stabilizer approved by the U.S. Food and Drug Administration (FDA) for the treatment of "manic episodes of manic-depressive illness" in patients aged 12 years and older?

    A. Valproate

    B. Carbamazepine

    C. Topiramate

    D. Lithium

    E. Lamotrigine

51. Methylphenidate and amphetamine are racemic mixtures which contain D- and L-enantiomers. Which is more pharmacologically active for methylphenidate?

    A. D-

    B. L-

    C. Neither; they are equally active

    D. Neither; the racemic mixture is ineffective until it is catabolized

52. Most orally administered psychotropic medications are absorbed primarily in which organ?

    A. Liver

    B. Colon

    C. Small intestine

    D. Stomach

53. Dopaminergic neurons from the substantia nigra project primarily to which brain areas?

    A. Caudate and putamen

    B. Nucleus accumbens and amygdala

    C. Frontal, cingulate, and entorhinal cortex

    D. Pituitary gland

54. All the following are dopaminergic modulating drugs that have been studied in the use of tics EXCEPT:

    A. Pergolide

    B. Bupropion

    C. Metoclopramide

    D. Tetrabenazine

55. In what year was electroconvulsive therapy (ECT) first administered?

    A. 1846

    B. 1902

    C. 1938

    D. 1955

56. Which of the following appears to lower serum clozapine levels?

    A. Smoking

    B. Caffeine

    C. Ciprofloxacin

    D. Erythromycin

57. Immediate-release preparations of bupropion are associated with seizures, particularly above which dosage?

    A. 100 mg daily

    B. 200 mg daily

    C. 300 mg daily

    D. 400 mg daily

58. In one epidemiological study, what percentage of preschoolers met criteria for an impairing DSM-IV disorder?

    A. 1%

    B. 2%

    C. 5%

    D. 12%

    E. 27%

59. Which of the following agents is the LEAST protein-bound?

    A. Fluoxetine

    B. Paroxetine

    C. Sertraline

    D. Citalopram

60. What is the evidence for the efficacy of elimination or restriction diets—diets that restrict certain food elements—in ADHD?

    A. The evidence is robust in favor of elimination diets

    B. The evidence is robust against elimination diets

    C. The evidence is promising

    D. Restriction diets have not been used in ADHD, only in autism

61. Psychopathy scores are correlated with which of the following traits?

    A. Younger age

    B. Male gender

    C. Suicide attempt

    D. All of the above

62. In what decade did bupropion emerge as a treatment for depression?

    A. 1940s

    B. 1960s

    C. 1980s

    D. 2000s

63. What occurs to alpha-2 receptors in the presence of endogenous alpha-2 agonists?

    A. Alpha-2 receptors disappear

    B. There is a net increase in alpha-2 receptors

    C. There is a net reduction in all three receptor subtypes

    D. Alpha-2 receptors are up-regulated

64. Where is the greatest concentration of serotonin found in the body?

    A. Brain and spinal cord

    B. Gastrointestinal lumen

    C. Platelets

    D. B and C

65. Olanzapine can attenuate insulin's effects on glucose and triglycerides in healthy normal-weight individuals:

    A. Related to the increase in body mass

    B. Independent of any change in body mass

    C. Related to the increase in fat percentage

    D. None of the above

66. Which of the following selective serotonin reuptake inhibitors (SSRIs) is FDA-approved for the treatment of childhood depression?

    A. Sertraline

    B. Citalopram

    C. Paroxetine

    D. Fluoxetine

Match the anatomic parts of a neuron with its respective function:

67. Dendrites

68. Cell body

69. Axon

70. Nerve terminals

    A. Provides a small area of close contact with dendrites of neighboring cells or a synapse

    B. Relay or output station of the neuron

    C. Creates a network of fibers providing the neuron with input from other cells

    D. Synthesis of all cell-specific receptors and enzymes needed for neurotransmitter production

71. Which of the following is the most consistent finding in structural MRI studies of pediatric major depressive disorder (MDD)?

    A. Reduced hypothalamic volume

    B. Reduced hippocampal volume

    C. Reduced frontal lobe volume

    D. Reduced temporal lobe volume

72. The Research Units on Pediatric Psychopharmacology (RUPP) Autism Network conducted its first drug study in 101 children and adolescents with autistic disorder who were assigned risperidone or placebo to assess improvement in what symptom?

    A. Depression

    B. Irritability

    C. Motor stereotypies

    D. Poor social reciprocity

    E. Psychosis

73. In the 7-point Clinical Global Impression-Improvement scale (CGI-I), what score generally demarcates a treatment "responder"?

    A. 1 or 2

    B. 3 or 4

    C. 5 or 6

    D. 7

74. A patient with which of the following disorders is most likely to respond to pharmacotherapy for obsessive-compulsive symptoms?

    A. OCD alone

    B. OCD and ADHD

    C. OCD and a tic disorder

    D. OCD and oppositional defiant disorder

75. Which of the following medications completely equilibrates across the placenta?

    A. Paroxetine

    B. Lithium

    C. Sertraline

    D. Fluoxetine

76. Which of the following is the best definition of obsessions?

    A. Thoughts that cannot be stopped, even with the help of counteracting actions

    B. Intrusive, repetitive thoughts, ideas, images, or impulses that are anxiety-provoking

    C. A single, driven desire

    D. Excessive daydreaming

77. All studies that have measured prolactin systematically in preschool children prescribed risperidone have reported:

    A. Undetectable prolactin changes

    B. Increased prolactin by 20- to 50-fold

    C. Increased prolactin by 3- to 5-fold

    D. Spurious increases related to tuberoinfundibular immaturity

78. The presence of a substance use disorder comorbid with bipolar disorder:

    A. Worsens the severity and course of both disorders

    B. Leads to a better outcome for the substance use disorder

    C. Improves the outcome of both disorders

    D. Reflects the most commonly occurring comorbid diagnoses in child psychiatry

79. Which of the following is the only synthetic melatonin receptor agonist with FDA approval for the treatment of insomnia?

    A. Zolpidem

    B. Ramelteon

    C. Eszopiclone

    D. Alprazolam

80. Stimulants have been used in the treatment of severe acute pain because they:

    A. Have independent analgesic effects

    B. Increase alertness, allowing greater opioid administration

    C. Potentiate the effects of analgesics

    D. All of the above

81. You evaluate an adolescent who has active bipolar disorder symptoms and a substance use disorder. Which of the following is advised?

    A. Start a mood stabilizer or antipsychotic after abstinence is achieved

    B. Start a mood stabilizer or antipsychotic with or without abstinence

    C. Recommend inpatient treatment for both

    D. Recommend electroconvulsive therapy

82. Some tertiary amine tricyclic antidepressants are metabolized to a secondary amine, such as imipramine, which is metabolized to:
    A. Clomipramine
    B. Trimipramine
    C. Nortriptyline
    D. Desipramine

83. Stimulants can lead to:
    A. Some reductions in expected growth velocity in height and weight
    B. Some reductions in expected growth velocity in height
    C. Some reductions in expected growth velocity in weight
    D. No expected reductions in growth velocity

84. Until the 1960s the doctor–patient relationship was dominated by:
    A. Autonomy
    B. Beneficence
    C. Paternalism
    D. Justice

85. Which of the following antipsychotics has evidence of superior effectiveness in managing aggression in pediatric and adult populations?
    A. Olanzapine
    B. Clozapine
    C. Aripiprazole
    D. Quetiapine

86. For youths taking psychotropic medications, which answer option is closest to the estimated percentage of those who are taking two or more psychotropics?
    A. 1% to 5%
    B. 5% to 20%
    C. 25% to 40%
    D. 60% to 75%
    E. Over 75%

87. Which of the following is an agonist of the GABA$_A$ receptor?
    A. Barbiturate
    B. Benzodiazepine
    C. Tricyclic antidepressant
    D. A and B

88. Which CYP enzyme is most relevant for the clearance of clozapine?
    A. 2D6
    B. 3A4
    C. 2B6
    D. 1A2

89. What are relative contraindications for the use of clonidine?
    A. Sinus tachycardia
    B. Sinus node and atrioventricular node disease
    C. Irritable bowel syndrome
    D. Seizure disorder

90. PET scan studies have demonstrated that acute alcohol intoxication reduces:
    A. Limbic system glucose metabolism
    B. Temporal lobe glucose metabolism
    C. Prefrontal glucose metabolism
    D. Parietal lobe glucose metabolism

91. The Child and Adolescent Bipolar Foundation (CABF) guidelines and American Academy of Child and Adolescent Psychiatry (AACAP) practice parameters for pediatric bipolar disorder recommend consideration of medication tapering or discontinuation after a successful remission for a minimum of how long?
    A. 6 months
    B. 8 months
    C. 12 to 24 months
    D. 24 to 36 months

92. **Which answer option best describes phase II metabolic reactions?**

    A. The formation of a link between the functionalized handle of a drug and a conjugate via a transferase

    B. The formation of a link between the functionalized handle of a drug and oxygen

    C. The formation of a link between the functionalized handle of a drug and cyclic adenosine monophosphate

    D. The formation of a link between the functionalized handle of a drug and a UGT (uridine diphosphate glucuronosyltransferase)

93. **Persons with Tourette's disorder may have a deficit in what area?**

    A. Sensory synesthesia

    B. Sensory discernment

    C. Sensory gating

    D. Sensory stimulation

94. **In effectiveness research, the inclusion criteria:**

    A. Are based on gender alone

    B. Are stringent

    C. Include a broad and diverse population likely to receive the treatment

    D. Are likely to include a homogeneous population

95. **What did a randomized controlled trial of clonidine show with respect to conduct disorder symptoms?**

    A. Symptoms improved

    B. Symptoms worsened

    C. Symptoms remained the same

    D. Symptoms improved only with combined SSRI treatment

96. **The stool softener polyethylene glycol-3350 is:**

    A. Not recommended for the treatment or prevention of pediatric constipation

    B. Recommended for the treatment or prevention of pediatric constipation

    C. Often contraindicated in the treatment or prevention of pediatric constipation

    D. Significantly absorbed by the colon

97. **Which of the following is the third leading cause of death in youths?**

    A. Suicides

    B. Motor vehicle accidents

    C. Homicides

    D. Cancers

98. **Which unilateral electrode placement at adequate suprathreshold doses is as effective as bilateral placement in electroconvulsive therapy (ECT)?**

    A. Right unilateral

    B. Left unilateral

    C. Right or left unilateral placement

    D. Unilateral ECT is not as effective as bilateral ECT

99. **Through the comparison of monozygotic twins and same-sex non-twin siblings prescribed clozapine, the heritability of clozapine-induced weight gain was calculated closest to which percentage?**

    A. 20%

    B. 50%

    C. 80%

    D. 100%

100. **Which two disorders or behaviors are commonly found with Tourette's disorder?**

    A. Attention-deficit/hyperactivity disorder and obsessive-compulsive disorder

    B. Major depressive disorder and oppositional defiant disorder

    C. Attention-deficit/hyperactivity disorder and separation anxiety disorder

    D. Anxiety disorder not otherwise specified and self-injurious behavior

101. **Which condition can be induced by exposure to substances that change respiratory patterns, such as sodium lactate, doxapram, and carbon dioxide?**

    A. Depression

    B. Panic attacks

    C. Generalized anxiety

    D. Dysthymia

102. **Gabapentin is approved for which indication(s)?**
   A. Bipolar I disorder
   B. Partial seizures
   C. Bipolar II disorder
   D. Post-herpetic neuralgia
   E. B and D

103. **Which of the following agents would warrant an ECG before starting treatment in a child?**
   A. Dextroamphetamine
   B. Ziprasidone
   C. Risperidone
   D. Methylphenidate
   E. Valproic acid

104. **Which agency has regulatory authority over the development and marketing of new drugs?**
   A. National Institutes of Health
   B. National Institute of Mental Health
   C. Centers for Medicare and Medicaid Services
   D. Food and Drug Administration

105. **Which of the following is NOT part of the basal ganglia?**
   A. Caudate
   B. Fornix
   C. Nucleus accumbens
   D. Globus pallidus

106. **All the following are a delivery mechanism for long-acting preparations of methylphenidate or amphetamine EXCEPT:**
   A. Wax-matrix
   B. Bead-filled capsule
   C. Osmotic release
   D. Pro-drug, cleavage of lysine
   E. Pulverized powder

107. **Which of the following would be reasons to use clonidine, guanfacine, or propranolol in posttraumatic stress disorder (PTSD)?**
   A. To reduce anxiety
   B. To reduce hyperarousal and re-experiencing phenomena
   C. To improve mood
   D. To reduce auditory hallucination-like symptoms

108. **When is rechallenge with clozapine not permitted?**
   A. WBC < 5000/mm^3 and/or ANC <2000/mm^3
   B. WBC <3000/mm^3 and/or ANC <2000/mm^3
   C. WBC <2500/mm^3 and/or ANC <1000/mm^3
   D. WBC <2000/mm^3 and/or ANC <1000/mm^3

109. **Which of the following conditions, like attention-deficit/hyperactivity disorder (ADHD), is associated with impulsive behaviors?**
   A. Oppositional defiant disorder
   B. Disruptive behavior disorder, not otherwise specified
   C. Selective mutism
   D. Lead poisoning

110. **Which of the following tricyclic antidepressant medications is associated with an increased risk of cardiotoxicity in prepubertal children?**
   A. Nortriptyline
   B. Desipramine
   C. Trimipramine
   D. Doxepin

111. **A 34-year-old man with treatment-resistant depression begins adjunct low-dose fluoxetine while being maintained on selegiline and soon becomes delirious. Which of the following is the most likely cause of the delirium?**
   A. Hypertensive crisis
   B. Acute dystonic reaction
   C. Serotonin syndrome
   D. Restless leg syndrome

112. **Which term describes how well a screening or diagnostic instrument will NOT detect a person who does NOT have the disorder and avoid false-positives?**
   A. Reliability
   B. Validity
   C. Sensitivity
   D. Specificity

113. **Bulimia nervosa is categorized into which two types?**
   A. Purging and non-purging
   B. Purging and restricting
   C. Binging and purging
   D. None of the above

114. **Which of the following is an accurate statement about products such as St. John's wort and flax-seed oil, which are classified as food products?**

    A. Manufacturers can advertise that they prevent disease

    B. Manufacturers can advertise that they treat disease

    C. Manufacturers can advertise that they cure disease

    D. Manufactures can advertise that they can influence the structure or function of the body

115. **Which of the following is an opiate antagonist that is used to reduce alcohol craving?**

    A. Buprenorphine

    B. L-alpha acetylmethadol (LAAM)

    C. Naloxone

    D. Naltrexone

116. **The mnemonic PECO stands for which of the following when formulating a clinical query for an evidence-based medicine search strategy?**

    A. Population, evidence, correlation, outcome

    B. Population, exposure, control, outcome

    C. Proband, exposure, concurrence, outcome

    D. Proband, evidence, condition, outlier

117. **Which of the following is an option used in clinical practice that has been shown to be effective for the treatment for ADHD?**

    A. Nortriptyline

    B. Paroxetine

    C. Mirtazapine

    D. Fluoxetine

118. **In cases of hyperprolactinemia, which common causes should be ruled out?**

    A. Pregnancy, hypothyroidism, renal failure

    B. Pregnancy, renal failure, acromegaly

    C. Acromegaly, depression, pregnancy

    D. Hypothyroidism, autism, Cushing's disease

119. **What is the rate-limiting step in the onset of action for benzodiazepines?**

    A. Absorption

    B. Serotonin receptor integrity

    C. P450 metabolism

    D. White matter density

120. **Which of the following is the most commonly used muscle relaxant in electroconvulsive therapy (ECT)?**

    A. Atracurium

    B. Succinylcholine

    C. Mivacurium

    D. None of the above

121. **What would be a recommended starting dosage of St. John's wort for an adolescent?**

    A. 100 mg daily

    B. 600 mg daily

    C. 150 mg three times daily

    D. 300 mg four times daily

122. **Which agent is most likely to increase prolactin levels?**

    A. Olanzapine

    B. Risperidone

    C. Ziprasidone

    D. Clozapine

    E. Aripiprazole

123. **A child presents with symptoms of obsessive-compulsive disorder (OCD) that warrant pharmacotherapy. The child also has comorbid attention-deficit/hyperactivity disorder (ADHD). Which of the following medication options might be used alone for both disorders?**

    A. Haloperidol

    B. Guanfacine

    C. Clomipramine

    D. Bupropion

124. **Most teens struggle to achieve age-appropriate autonomy while trying to accept their psychiatric illness. This often leads to:**

    A. Insight

    B. Treatment non-adherence

    C. Family collusion

    D. Running away

125. **In a clinical trial, what is a type II error?**

    A. Rejecting the null hypothesis when the difference is in fact due to chance

    B. Failing to reject the null hypothesis when there is a real difference between treatment groups

    C. The ability to detect a difference due to chance

    D. The ability to detect a difference due to real effect

126. **Which statement describes renal drug elimination efficiency in children compared to adults?**

    A. More efficient

    B. Equally efficient

    C. Less efficient

    D. None of the above

127. **Youths with bipolar disorder take a longer time to recover when they present with which of the following initial mood episodes?**

    A. Manic episode

    B. Major depressive episode

    C. Mixed episode

    D. None of the above

128. **Longitudinal studies suggest that treatment for attention-deficit/hyperactivity disorder (ADHD):**

    A. Increases the risk for substance use disorders in adulthood

    B. Increases the risk for antisocial personality disorder

    C. Has little effect on the eventual risk of substance use in adulthood

    D. Increases the risk for conduct disorder

129. **What are phase III trials?**

    A. Post-marketing studies to delineate additional information, including the drug's risks, benefits, and optimal use

    B. Initial studies to determine the metabolism and pharmacologic actions of drugs in humans and the side effects associated with increasing doses, and to gain early evidence of effectiveness; may include healthy participants and/or patients

    C. Controlled clinical studies conducted to evaluate the effectiveness of the drug for a particular indication(s) in patients with the disease or condition under study and to determine the common short-term side effects and risks

    D. Expanded controlled and uncontrolled trials after preliminary evidence suggesting effectiveness of the drug has been obtained; intended to gather additional information to evaluate the overall benefit/risk relationship of the drug and provide an adequate basis for physician labeling

130. **Cardiac side effects of lithium treatment include all the following EXCEPT:**

    A. Conduction delays

    B. Ventricular tachycardia

    C. Sinus arrhythmia

    D. Premature ventricular contractions

    E. First-degree atrioventricular block

131. ***In utero* exposure to what medication was associated with reduced newborn behavioral response to pain induced by the phenylketonuria (PKU) heel lance?**

    A. Serotonin reuptake inhibitors

    B. Benzodiazepines

    C. Atypical antipsychotics

    D. Lithium

132. **Which TWO of the following are the common side effects of transcranial magnetic stimulation (TMS) as reported by adult patients?**

    A. Headache

    B. Epistaxis

    C. Scalp pain

    D. Seizures

133. Carbamazepine is an anticonvulsant agent structurally similar to:
    A. Lamotrigine
    B. Valproic acid
    C. Lithium
    D. Imipramine

134. Data from the Medical Expenditure Panel Survey indicate that the annual rate of outpatient treatment, whether therapy or medications, for depression among children and adolescents is:
    A. 1 per 100 persons
    B. 15 per 100 persons
    C. 25 per 100 persons
    D. >30 per 100 persons

135. The data for atypical antipsychotics in adults with delirium best support the use of:
    A. Quetiapine and aripiprazole
    B. Olanzapine and risperidone
    C. Clozapine and risperidone
    D. Quetiapine and ziprasidone

136. Which of the following endogenous substances has been found to help the availability and utilization of energy critical for the fight-or-flight response to stress?
    A. Serotonin
    B. Glucocorticoids
    C. Opioids
    D. Glutamate

137. All females treated with valproate should have a baseline assessment of menstrual cycle patterns, as well as continued monitoring of menstrual irregularities, weight gain, hirsutism, and acne, due to the possible increased risk of:
    A. Liver dysfunction
    B. Polycystic ovarian syndrome (PCOS)
    C. Hyperammonemia
    D. Hypothyroidism
    E. Hyperparathyroidism

138. What is the organ of origin for the hormone ghrelin?
    A. Adipose tissue
    B. Gastrointestinal tract
    C. Hypothalamus
    D. Kidney

139. The Multimodal Treatment of ADHD (MTA) study found that high-quality medication management consisted of monthly visits that attended not only to medication benefits and side effects but also to all of the following elements EXCEPT:
    A. Checks on adherence and tolerability
    B. Consideration of unconscious determinants of behavior
    C. Progress in school
    D. State of relationships with peers and family

140. During what period of gestation does cardiogenesis occur?
    A. Day 1 to 35
    B. Day 15 to 56
    C. Day 60 to 93
    D. Day 93 to 120

141. What kind of antidepressant mechanism is more prominent in duloxetine and venlafaxine at higher doses?
    A. Serotonin reuptake inhibition
    B. Norepinephrine reuptake inhibition
    C. Dopamine reuptake inhibition
    D. Glutamate inhibition

142. In a child exposed to trauma, which of the following is the most common co-occurring disorder?
    A. Major depressive episode
    B. Another anxiety disorder
    C. Psychotic disorder, not otherwise specified
    D. Bipolar disorder

143. Which of the following selective serotonin reuptake inhibitors (SSRIs) has the highest risk ratio for suicidal thinking and behavior in children?

    A. Paroxetine

    B. Fluoxetine

    C. Sertraline

    D. Escitalopram

    E. The risk is equal

144. Benzodiazepines might be effective in a patient to treat which of the following?

    A. Re-experiencing

    B. Insomnia

    C. Avoidance

    D. Numbing

145. The following are elements of informed consent as outlined by the American Academy of Pediatrics Committee on Bioethics, following the thinking of ethicist and forensic psychiatrist Paul Appelbaum, EXCEPT:

    A. Information: patients should have, in everyday, understandable language, explanations of the medical problem, any additional diagnostic procedures recommended, proposed treatments, the likelihood of treatment success, as well as the potential risks and benefits of the recommended treatments, alternative treatments, and no treatment

    B. Assessment of the patient or decision-maker's understanding of the information provided

    C. An assessment of the patient or the surrogate decision-maker's capacity to make medical decisions about the care of the child or adolescent

    D. The freedom of the patient and/or decision-maker to make choices and decisions without being manipulated or coerced in any way

    E. Documentation of the discussion with the patient or decision-maker in the affirmative or negative

146. Levels of skin conductance or electrodermal responding represent the electrical activity of skin and reflect the activity of which system?

    A. Hypothalamic-pituitary-adrenal (HPA) axis

    B. Sympathetic nervous system

    C. Parasympathetic nervous system

    D. Motor reflex arc

147. All the following are true EXCEPT:

    A. Human beings do not learn to aggress, they learn <u>not</u> to aggress

    B. 25% of all daycare interactions involve aggression

    C. Aggression is maladaptive

    D. Aggression is sanctioned by society for self-defense or warfare

148. All the following are general medication side effect rating scales EXCEPT:

    A. Monitoring of Side Effects System (MOSES)

    B. Abnormal Involuntary Movement Scale (AIMS)

    C. Side Effects Rating Scale

    D. Safety Monitoring Uniform Report Form (SMURF)

149. Which of the following medications, when initiated prior to puberty, has been reported to cause pubertal arrest?

    A. Fluoxetine

    B. Imipramine

    C. Valproic acid

    D. Dextroamphetamine

150. One of the principal roles of neuropsychological testing in children with attention-deficit/hyperactivity disorder (ADHD) is to:

    A. Support the diagnosis of ADHD

    B. Determine the diagnosis of ADHD

    C. Document comorbid learning disorders

    D. Obtain disability payments

151. Between 1996 and 2001, the prescriptions of antipsychotic agents for preschool children increased to what degree?

    A. Marginal statistical increase

    B. Two-fold

    C. Three-fold

    D. More than five-fold

152. Which of the following is an effect of serotonin reuptake inhibitors that is especially relevant to consider when consulting on patients with thrombocytopenia or coagulopathies?

    A. Interference with platelet aggregation

    B. Nausea

    C. Paresthesias

    D. Hyperhidrosis

153. Compared with adults, the risk of children less than 16 years old developing a serious rash on lamotrigine treatment is:

    A. Less

    B. The same

    C. 2 times greater

    D. 3 times greater

    E. 5 times greater

154. The mortality rate associated with electroconvulsive therapy (ECT) is:

    A. 1 in 2000 treatments

    B. 1 in 40,000 treatments

    C. 1 in 80,000 treatments

    D. 1 in 200,000 treatments

155. Benzodiazepines act throughout the central nervous system. Their anxiolytic effects are attributed to their action upon:

    A. Limbic and cortical areas

    B. Spinal cord

    C. Brain stem

    D. Reticular formation

156. Retrospective and prospective studies suggest that the diagnosis of generalized anxiety disorder (GAD) during adolescence strongly predicts which condition during adulthood?

    A. Generalized anxiety

    B. Major depression

    C. Bipolar disorder

    D. Dysthymia

157. What is the developmental pattern of growth of the amygdala in typically developing children?

    A. Substantial increase in volume from 7.5 to 18.5 years old

    B. Substantial decrease in volume from 7.5 to 18.5 years old

    C. No change in volume after 7.5 years old

    D. No change in volume after birth

158. Testing the efficacy of a pharmacological treatment against an established treatment is called:

    A. An inferiority trial

    B. Active control equivalency study

    C. A superiority trial

    D. A & B

    E. B & C

159. Prior to starting medications, the main reason for a review of pre-existing physical complaints, sleep and eating habits, gastrointestinal and urological function, energy level, psychiatric symptoms, and emotional regulation is to:

    A. Monitor for symptoms that occur or worsen after the start of treatment

    B. Satisfy Medicaid requirements

    C. Avoid legal liability

    D. Reassure the parents

160. Which of the following describes the process of mechanism-based inhibition?

    A. Tight binding to CYP docking site without destruction of the site

    B. Reversible binding to CYP docking site

    C. Tight binding to CYP docking site with destruction of the site

    D. High-affinity binding to CYP docking site

161. Which serious side effect is associated with topiramate treatment?

    A. Hyperthermia

    B. Stevens-Johnson syndrome

    C. Cognitive Impairment

    D. Weight gain

    E. A and C

162. Which of the following is the only approach associated with long-term cure of pediatric nocturnal enuresis?

    A. Imipramine

    B. Bell-and-pad device

    C. DDAVP

    D. Making the child wash and change the bedclothes

163. When treating a child with obsessive-compulsive disorder (OCD) who has not been responsive to weekly cognitive behavioral therapy (CBT), an SSRI medication should be considered after:

    A. 1 to 2 weeks

    B. 2 to 4 weeks

    C. 4 to 6 weeks

    D. 8 to 12 weeks

164. What percentage of children with separation anxiety disorder will manifest symptoms of a psychiatric disorder in adulthood?

    A. 2%

    B. 5%

    C. 10%

    D. 33%

165. Clonidine and guanfacine work principally through which of the following?

    A. Alpha-2 agonism

    B. Alpha-2 antagonism

    C. Beta-2 agonism

    D. Beta-1 antagonism

166. Autism is more common in males than females by a ratio of:

    A. 1.5 to 1

    B. 2 to 1

    C. 4 to 1

    D. 10 to 1

    E. None of the above

167. Which of the following allowed pharmaceutical sponsors the possibility of gaining an additional 6 months of market exclusivity (freedom from generic competition) for their drugs?

    A. Pediatric Research Equity Act (PREA) of 2003

    B. Pediatric Use subsection under the Precautions section of labeling in 1979

    C. Food and Drug Administration Modernization Act (FDAMA) of 1997

    D. Food and Drug Administration Amendments Act (FDAAA) of 2007

    E. Pediatric Rule of 1998

168. What is the primary indication of electroconvulsive therapy (ECT) in adolescents?

    A. Schizophrenia

    B. Depressive symptoms

    C. Manic symptoms

    D. B & C

169. Although discovered in the 1970s, FDA approval of bupropion was delayed until 1989 due to which concern?

    A. QT prolongation at higher doses

    B. Increased risk of seizures in patients with bulimia

    C. Hypertension at higher doses

    D. B and C

170. Which of the following sedating medications is the most commonly prescribed in pediatric practice?

    A. Antihistamine

    B. Melatonin

    C. Clonidine

    D. Zaleplon

    E. Klonopin

171. A recent literature review found that melatonin improves what aspect of sleep?

    A. Sleep onset latency

    B. Middle-of-the-night awakening

    C. Early-morning awakening

    D. All of the above

172. What methods are suitable for discovering the long-term effects of medications on intelligence, personality, and other more subtle aspects of human behavior?

    A. Registry data

    B. Case control studies

    C. Long-term controlled studies

    D. Cohort studies

173. Which of the following has been associated with a decreased response to psychopharmacological treatment in pediatric anxiety?

    A. Younger age

    B. Milder symptoms

    C. Parental depression

    D. Extroversion

For the following questions, match the drug with the correct FDA labeling for children and/or adolescents. A drug may have more than one correct corresponding answer option, or an answer option may correspond to more than one drug

174. Clomipramine

175. Pimozide

176. Haloperidol

177. Imipramine

178. Doxepin

    A. Labeling indicates use for Tourette's disorder

    B. Approved for obsessive-compulsive disorder

    C. Approved for enuresis

    D. Approved for "psychoneurosis" with labeling suggesting that safety and effectiveness in patients below the age of 12 years have not been established

179. Which of the following agents has been most studied in anorexia nervosa?

    A. Risperidone

    B. Quetiapine

    C. Aripiprazole

    D. Olanzapine

180. Which of the following is LEAST likely to be an important focus of research needed to help expand the currently available pharmacoepidemiological data about prescription patterns?

    A. The safety and efficacy of psychotropic medications

    B. The extent to which evidence-based practices are being implemented

    C. Examining prescription patterns coupled to independently determined diagnoses rather than relying on physician report

    D. The extent to which physicians consult with one another about cases

    E. Prevalence of medication use in the presence or absence of other types of treatment

181. A controlled trial of girls with anorexia nervosa who were randomized to inpatient treatment, specialized outpatient treatment, or general child and adolescent mental health services found which of the following?

    A. Inpatient treatment led to better outcomes

    B. Specialized outpatient treatment led to better outcomes

    C. Specialized outpatient treatment and general outpatient centers had the same outcomes

    D. Specialized outpatient treatment led to the worst outcomes

182. Which of the following medications has a controlled trial showing effectiveness compared to placebo in reducing binging and purging episodes?

    A. Lithium

    B. Topiramate

    C. Lamotrigine

    D. Depakote

183. Which is the most frequent co-occurring diagnosis with childhood-onset schizophrenia?

    A. Generalized anxiety disorder

    B. Obsessive-compulsive disorder

    C. A depressive disorder

    D. Attention-deficit/hyperactivity disorder

184. What percentage of cases in obsessive-compulsive disorder (OCD) is familial?

    A. 10%

    B. 25%

    C. 50%

    D. 75%

185. A recent study of self-reports of physical violence during early childhood to early adulthood found which TWO factors were inversely associated with a high frequency of physical violence?

    A. Executive functioning

    B. Nonverbal IQ

    C. Verbal IQ

    D. Visual-motor integration

186. Selective serotonin reuptake inhibitors (SSRIs) exert their effects through what mechanism primarily?

　　A. Postsynaptic inhibition of norepinephrine cross-talk receptors

　　B. Postsynaptic inhibition of serotonin reuptake

　　C. Presynaptic inhibition of serotonin reuptake

　　D. Presynaptic inhibition of tyrosine uptake

187. Which of the following is an accurate statement about binge eating disorder in adults and selective serotonin reuptake inhibitors (SSRIs)?

　　A. SSRIs are equal to placebo in reducing binge attacks

　　B. SSRIs are superior to placebo in reducing binge attacks

　　C. SSRIs are inferior to placebo in reducing binge attacks

　　D. There are no controlled trials of SSRIs evaluating effectiveness in binge eating

188. Which country has the lowest prevalence of stimulant use among the following countries?

　　A. Australia

　　B. Germany

　　C. Canada

　　D. United States

189. Monoamine oxidase-A (MAO-A) is predominantly found where in the body?

　　A. Intestines

　　B. CNS

　　C. Sympathetic nerve terminals

　　D. A and C

190. Which of the following is a commonly used scale for obsessive-compulsive disorder (OCD) in children?

　　A. Yale-Brown Obsessive Compulsive Scale, children's version

　　B. Global Assessment of Function Scale

　　C. Self-report for Childhood Anxiety Related Disorders

　　D. The Child and Adolescent Psychiatry Screen

191. What is the maximum one-time dose for the immediate-release formulation of bupropion in adults?

　　A. 75 mg

　　B. 150 mg

　　C. 300 mg

　　D. 450 mg

192. A 15-year-old girl on lithium and another medication develops nausea, vomiting, and slurred speech. Which of the following increases the risk of lithium toxicity?

　　A. Quetiapine

　　B. Carbamazepine

　　C. Sertraline

　　D. Librium

193. To diagnose a child with major depressive disorder (MDD), there must be the presence of a persistent depressed or irritable mood or marked anhedonia for at least what duration of time?

　　A. 2 days

　　B. 2 weeks

　　C. 2 months

　　D. 3 months

194. Which term describes the common-sense applicability of a screening instrument in asking about symptoms for a disorder it is intending to screen for?

　　A. Face validity

　　B. Content validity

　　C. Positive predictive power

　　D. Negative predictive power

195. The FDA has regulatory oversight over all the following EXCEPT:

　　A. Drugs

　　B. Ethanol

　　C. Biological treatments

　　D. Medical devices

Match the substance dependence disorder with the appropriate FDA-approved medication for treatment (more than one answer is possible)

196. Alcohol dependence

197. Nicotine dependence

198. Opiate dependence

    A.   Acamprosate

    B.   Bupropion

    C.   Disulfiram

    D.   Methadone

    E.   Naltrexone

    F.   Buprenorphine

    G.   Varenicline

    H.   Nicotine replacement

199. According to the American Academy of Child and Adolescent Psychiatry, conflict of interest is best described as:

    A.   Two or more interests

    B.   The risk that patient care or patient welfare will be compromised by a secondary interest

    C.   The secondary gain that may drive a clinician to act, either consciously, subconsciously, or unconsciously, and that is not in the patient's best interest

    D.   Two opposing views of the benefits and/or risks of treatment

200. **Pregabalin does which of the following?**

    A.   Reduces glutamate

    B.   Increases norepinephrine

    C.   Increases substance P

    D.   Methylates brain-derived neurotrophic factor (BDNF)

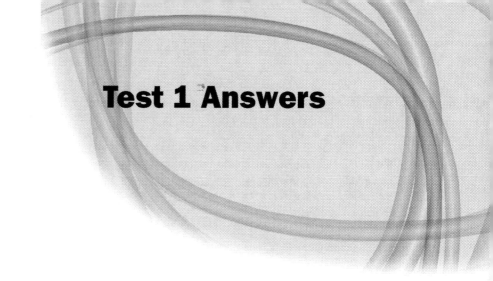

Test 1 Answers

1. Answer: B

Risperidone and ziprasidone are likely to have the greatest risk for EPS among the second-generation antipsychotics. (Chap. 37)

2. Answer: D

Higher-SES youths are prescribed more psychotropic medications than their lower-SES counterparts. However, youths with impairment (e.g., receiving special education services, disability income) and those with social deprivation (e.g., foster care youths) are commonly prescribed more psychotropic medications in the United States and elsewhere. (Chap. 54)

3. Answer: D

Non-adherence for asthma, diabetes, and epilepsy is common. The list also includes juvenile rheumatoid arthritis and transplantation. (Chap. 3)

4. Answer: A

The process of hippocampal atrophy and neurogenesis may be related to the pathophysiology of depression, although it is likely that only some of the therapeutic actions of antidepressants are dependent on hippocampal neurogenesis. (Chap. 1)

5. Answer: B

Those listed are but a few of a variety of short-acting, intermediate-acting, and long-acting agents. (Chap. 31)

6. Answer: D

Methylphenidate and risperidone have the most data in reducing aggression. (Chap. 47)

7. Answer: E

Valproic acid has been used to treat epilepsy, bipolar disorder, migraine headaches, and schizophrenia. It has less commonly been used to treat major depression. (Chap. 22)

8. Answer: D

Desipramine selectively blocks the norepinephrine transporter. (Chap. 2)

9. Answer: D

One-third of the thirty to forty thousand protein-coding protein genes are expressed in the central nervous system. The intrinsic complexity of the central nervous system, both structurally and functionally, appears to account for this great share of the human genome dedicated to it. (Chap. 1)

10. Answer: C

The majority of children presenting with hallucinations are likely to have an affective disorder and not early-onset schizophrenia spectrum disorder (EOSS). (Chap. 37)

11. Answer: D

Moreover, maintenance treatment is recommended for adults with difficult-to-treat depressive episodes and those with second episodes associated with severe impairment. (Chap. 32)

12. Answer: D

The inhibition constant, K_i, is an indicator of how potent an inhibitor is, with lower values representing greater inhibition. (Chap. 4)

13. Answer: A

The TDT is considered the gold standard in the detection of associations. (Chap. 6)

14. Answer: B

The cerebellum processes motor and cognitive information. (Chap. 2)

15. Answer: D

Animal models suggested buspirone might have anxiolytic properties, and it was developed as such after clinical trials showed little antipsychotic effect. (Chap. 24)

16. Answer: C

Males are two to four times more likely to receive a psychotropic than females. (Chap. 49)

17. Answer: A

TCAs were initially used as hypnotics and antiparkinsonian agents. The discovery that TCAs (imipramine) improve mood occurred in 1954. (Chap. 21)

18. Answer: A

Group cognitive therapy has enough evidence to say it is probably efficacious. Individual cognitive therapy has the best evidence. The "Coping Cat" by Kendall is an example of a CBT manual, with child and adolescent versions. (Chap. 34)

19. Answer: C

In a mixed episode of bipolar disorder, symptoms of both mania and depression are present without either predominating. (Chap. 33)

20. Answer: A

The second-generation antipsychotics are associated with a lower occurrence of NMS than the first-generation antipsychotics—or at least the SGAs are associated with a more benign course. Bromocriptine seemed to reduce the duration of symptoms, whereas dantrolene did not. (Chap. 23)

21. Answer: B

While children with behavioral inhibition face a high risk for a variety of childhood anxiety disorders, the risk is specific for social phobia by adolescence. (Chap. 10)

22. Answer: C

Fluoxetine is FDA-approved for MDD (ages 8 and older) and OCD (ages 7 and older) in pediatric populations. Fluoxetine also has positive RCTs for selective mutism, generalized anxiety disorder, and repetitive behaviors in pervasive developmental disorders (citalopram, another SSRI, has shown no effect for repetitive behaviors). (Chap. 20)

23. Answer: B

Kava-kava, an herbal sleep aid, has been associated with hepatotoxicity. (Chap. 46)

24. Answer: D

Slightly more than one-third of the children studied displayed hypersexuality, which was less commonly found than increased energy, distractibility, and pressured speech. (Chap. 33)

25. Answer: C

The continuation phase lasts for 6 to 12 months and follows the acute phase of treatment for MDD which is the initial 3 months. (Chap. 32)

26. Answer: B

Clonidine has alpha 2a, 2b, and 2c properties, and the role of 2b appears to be restricted to cardiovascular function. (Chap. 19)

27. Answer: A

First-order is linear kinetics; zero-order kinetics is nonlinear. (Chap. 3)

28. Answer: B

The ability of rating scales to determine treatment effects is contingent on the construct validity (ability to measure specifically the intended psychopathology) and inter-rater reliability (consistency of measurement across clinicians). (Chap. 50)

29. Answer: A

Studies have shown an increase in blood pressure of 3–4 mm and an increase in heart rate of 1–2 beats per minute. (Chap. 43)

30. Answer: D

Dopamine D2 receptor antagonism in the tuberoinfundibular pathway leads to hyperprolactinemia. (Chap. 23)

31. Answer: D

A full-term newborn has about 70% total body water; adult values of 55% are reached by 12 years. (Chap. 3)

32. Answer: B

Antipsychotics are prescribed more often to treat aggression in children and adolescents than psychotic symptoms. (Chap. 42)

33. Answer: C

The estimated prevalence of Tourette's disorder is 3 to 10 per 1000. (Chap. 36)

34. Answer: D

In a chart review of 172 pediatric patients receiving clozapine, the cumulative 1-year probability of an initial adverse hematologic event was 16%; most youths were successfully rechallenged, with only 8 discontinuing because of neutropenia (n = 7) or agranulocytosis (n = 1). (Chap. 23)

35. Answer: D

The antagonism of presynaptic alpha-2 receptors increases norepinephrine concentrations, and the antagonism of the specified serotonin receptors decreases gastrointestinal and sexual adverse effects of increased serotonin. (Chap. 21)

36. Answer: D

Increases in total body water and the glomerular filtration rate during pregnancy lead to reduction of lithium levels during pregnancy. (Chap. 44)

37. Answer: C

In adults the half-life for diphenhydramine is 4 hours; for hydroxyzine it is 20 hours. In children the half-life is decreased for both diphenhydramine and hydroxyzine, with a half-life of 7 hours for hydroxyzine. (Chap. 24)

38. Answer: B

Studies aimed at examining the pharmacokinetics and toxicity of new treatments are called phase I trials. (Chap. 50)

39. Answer: C

These are findings of central serotonin syndrome, which can have similarities to NMS and catatonia. CSS rarely occurs with monotherapy but is a risk when a pro-serotonergic agent is added to another. (Chap. 4)

40. Answer: C

The FDA had contraindicated the use of stimulants in tic disorders and the labeling continues to do so. However, recent data indicate stimulants can be used safely in tic disorders, with methylphenidate perhaps better tolerated than amphetamine. (Chap. 36)

41. Answer: A

Carlsson observed that OCD can be considered a hyperglutamatergic syndrome. There appears to be a reciprocal relationship between glutamate and serotonin. Augmentation trials of glutamate modulating agents have been completed in adults with positive preliminary results. (Chap. 11)

42. Answer: A

The typical antipsychotics have been the most studied in tic disorders and have the best evidence for efficacy. The atypical agents are often preferred because of their side effect profile. (Chap. 36)

43. Answer: B

Anterograde amnesia is seen most commonly with intravenous administration of benzodiazepines, although this may also happen with oral administration. (Chap. 24)

44. Answer: D

Gabapentin does not affect glutamatergic function. (Chap. 38)

45. Answer: A

The half-life of extended-release and immediate-release guanfacine is similar. The primary rate of difference is the prolonged rate of dissolution of the extended-release formulation because of incorporation of polymers and organic acids. The more gradual and prolonged onset provides the extended duration of behavioral effects and allows a once-a-day dosing strategy. (Chap. 19)

46. Answer: C

All the options might or might not be reasonable measures to take, but the mandated obligation is to report the abuse to child protective services. (Chap. 27)

47. Answer: C

Zolpidem is mostly metabolized through CYP3A4 and less so through CYP2D6; therefore, inhibitors of 3A4 and 2D6 may slow elimination of zolpidem. (Chap. 24)

48. Answer: C

Buspirone is an agonist at 5-HT$_{1A}$. (Chap. 42)

49. Answer: B

Family involvement is one of the strongest predictors of adolescent outcome. (Chap. 41)

50. Answer: D

Lithium was first used over 40 years ago to treat pediatric bipolar disorder. (Chap. 22)

51. Answer: A

The D- enantiomer is more pharmacologically active in MPH. (Chap. 18)

52. Answer: C

Most oral psychotropic medications are absorbed in the small intestine. (Chap. 3)

53. Answer: A

Dopaminergic neurons from the substantia nigra are called A9 neurons and project to the caudate and putamen. (Chap. 2)

54. Answer: B

Bupropion has some dopaminergic action but has not been studied in tic disorders; its mechanism of action does not make it a good candidate for tic disorders. Pergolide was removed from the market in 2007 because it led to heart problems. (Chap. 36)

55. Answer: C

ECT was first administered in 1938 to a 39-year-old man with schizophrenia. (Chap. 26)

56. Answer: A

Clozapine serum levels may increase with smoking cessation. (Chap. 37)

57. Answer: D

The associated risk for seizures with bupropion has been shown to be elevated with rapidly increasing dosages and possibly in patients with bulimia. (Chap. 32)

58. Answer: D

12% of preschoolers met criteria for a DSM-IV disorder in an epidemiological study by Egger and Angold (2006). (Chap. 45)

59. Answer: D

Administration of highly protein-bound SSRIs like fluoxetine, sertraline, and paroxetine may be a concern when other highly protein-bound medications are administered, such as warfarin, diazepam, or propranolol. (Chap. 20)

60. Answer: C

The use of artificial colors and flavors and refined sugars has been linked by some to ADHD. Trials have produced conflicting results with more recent evidence promising. (The textbook does not reflect newer data). (Chap. 25)

61. Answer: D

Psychopathy scores also correlated with violent behavior, imprisonment, homelessness, and drug dependence. (Chap. 15)

62. Answer: C

Bupropion emerged as a treatment for depression in the 1980s. (Chap. 21)

63. Answer: C

In the presence of endogenous alpha agonists, adrenergic receptors are reduced, such that down-regulation to 50% of pretreatment values occurs after approximately 2.5 hours. Interestingly, the alpha-2a receptor subtype requires more agonist to be down-regulated than the b or c receptor subtypes; this could explain the clinically observed rapid tolerance to adverse effects but not therapeutic effects, given that 2a is thought to be the clinically relevant subtype. (Chap. 19)

64. Answer: D

Serotonin or 5-hydroxytryptamine (5-HT) plays a critical role in peristalsis and hemostasis. (Chap. 2)

65. Answer: B

Olanzapine blunts insulin's effects independent of any change in body mass or fat. (Chap. 37)

66. Answer: D

Fluoxetine is approved for child and adolescent depression. (Chap. 32)

67–70. Answer
67-C; 68-D; 69-B; 70-A. (Chap. 2)

71. Answer: B

Reduced hippocampal volume. Another consistent finding among children and adolescents with MDD is larger pituitary gland volumes compared to case-matched controls. (Chap. 9)

72. Answer: B

Irritability included aggression, self-injury, tantrums, and quickly changing moods. Risperidone treatment resulted in 69% of subjects being categorized as treatment responders, compared with 12% of those who received placebo. (Chap. 38)

73. Answer: A

In the CGI-I, 1 is very much improved, 2 much improved, 3 minimally improved, 4 no change, 5 minimally worse, 6 much worse, 7 very much worse. (Chap. 28)

74. Answer: A

The presence of certain co-occurring disorders reduces the likelihood of response to treatment. (Chap. 35)

75. Answer: B

In contrast to the incomplete placental passage of SSRIs, lithium completely equilibrates across the placenta, exposing the fetus to maternal plasma concentrations of lithium. (Chap. 44)

76. Answer: B

Obsessions are intrusive, repetitive thoughts, ideas, images, or impulses that are worries. (Chap. 35)

77. Answer: C

Prolactin elevations averaged 3- to 5-fold over the normal range of 10 ng/mL, but children remained asymptomatic. (Chap. 45)

78. Answer: A

The presence of substance abuse disorder comorbid with bipolar disorder worsens the severity and course of both disorders. (Chap. 33)

79. Answer: B

Ramelteon is a synthetic melatonin receptor agonist. (Chap. 46)

80. Answer: D

Stimulants have been used in the treatment of severe, acute pain, such as in sickle cell crisis, because they potentiate other analgesics, increase alertness with opioid use, and have independent analgesic effects. (Chap. 43)

81. Answer: B

The data indicate that mood stabilizers (lithium and valproic acid) may in fact reduce substance use in patients with bipolar disorder; given active symptomatology, waiting for abstinence is not required. Lithium should likely be used as a second-line treatment, given the narrower therapeutic index. An inpatient stay could be required depending on other factors, but this should not affect the decision to start a mood stabilizer. (Chap. 41)

82. Answer: D

Imipramine is metabolized to desipramine. (Chap. 21)

83. Answer: A

Stimulants can lead to some reductions in expected growth velocity in height and weight, but these reductions, on average, are small, attenuate with time, and do not cause a greater proportion of children to become extremely short or thin. However, children on stimulants should be monitored for growth progression and evaluated further if growth velocity declines unduly. (Chap. 31)

84. Answer: C

The doctor–patient relationship was largely paternalistic until recent times. At its best, paternalism denotes kindly, parental attitudes and care of individuals in which the clinician acts benevolently with the patient's best interest at heart. However, when taken to an extreme, paternalism may restrict individual autonomy and may be prejudicial, unfair, and even harmful. (Chap. 52)

85. Answer: B

There is evidence for clozapine's superiority over other antipsychotics in managing aggression in pediatric and adult populations. (Chap. 37)

86. Answer: C

The percentage of youths taking two or more psychotropics has been estimated to range from 25% to 40%, although others have found higher figures. (Chap. 4)

87. Answer: D

Both benzodiazepines and barbiturates are agonists of $GABA_A$. (Chap. 2)

88. Answer: D

Clozapine is cleared by 1A2. (Chap. 23)

89. Answer: B

Sinus node and atrioventricular node disease are relative contraindications as they can present with syncope and bradycardia; the latter can be exacerbated by alpha agonists. (Chap. 19)

90. Answer: C

Cognitive interference, among other mechanisms, appears to contribute to the pro-aggressive effects of alcohol. (Chap. 15)

91. Answer: C

Practice parameters have recommended considering tapering medication after 12 to 24 months of remission. (Chap. 33)

92. Answer: A

The most abundant conjugate in phase II reactions is glucuronic acid. UGTs serve to "hook up" the conjugate to the handle but are not the conjugate themselves. (Chap. 4)

93. Answer: C

Persons with Tourette's disorder appear to have a deficit in sensory gating. (Chap. 12)

94. Answer: C

Effectiveness research usually examines the effect of a treatment in usual practice conditions, whereas efficacy research is usually focused on the effect of treatment in ideal conditions and will include stringent inclusion criteria, a control group, and a focus on symptom outcome measures. The distinction between efficacy and effectiveness research can be a subtle one, and the interpretation of meaning also varies. (Chap. 50)

95. Answer: A

Symptoms improved on clonidine for conduct disorder. One study showed that clonidine combined with stimulants reduced the irritability and headaches associated with stimulant treatment. (Chap. 47)

96. Answer: B

Polyethylene glycol-3350 is not absorbed and is rarely contraindicated in children, and stool softeners are a central component in the treatment and prevention of pediatric constipation. (Chap. 48)

97. Answer: A

Suicide is the third leading cause of death in youths. (Chap. 9)

98. Answer: A

Right unilateral ECT is as effective as bilateral ECT and is likely to produce less severe cognitive effects. (Chap. 26)

99. Answer: C

The heritability appears to be 80%. The high degree of heritability suggests that genetic factors influence the variability of weight gain among users of antipsychotics. (Chap. 6)

100. Answer: A

ADHD is present in 70% and OCD symptoms in 40% to 50% of patients. (Chap. 12)

101. Answer: B

This induction of panic attacks indicates evidence of a biological correlate for clinical anxiety. (Chap. 10)

102. Answer: E

Gabapentin is FDA-approved for post-herpetic neuralgia in adults and for partial seizures in patients 12 years and older. (Chap. 22)

103. Answer: B

There is a consensus that use of TCAs, pimozide, thioridazine, and ziprasidone warrants an ECG. The American Academy of Pediatrics and the American Heart Association have concluded it is not necessary to obtain an ECG before ADHD pharmacotherapy, but one may be warranted depending on the cardiovascular history of the child and/ or family. (Chap. 27)

104. Answer: D

The FDA has regulatory authority over the development and marketing of new drugs. (Chap. 51)

105. Answer: B

The fornix is not part of the basal ganglia. The basal ganglia also consist of the putamen and the substantia nigra. (Chap. 11)

106. Answer: E

Pulverized powder is not a delivery mechanism for stimulants. (Chap. 18)

107. Answer: B

Adrenergic agents such as the alpha-2 agonists, clonidine, and guanfacine and the beta-antagonist propranolol can reduce sympathetic arousal. (Chap. 39)

108. Answer: D

If the WBC is less than $2000/mm^3$ and/or the ANC is less than $1000/mm^3$, clozapine is to be discontinued and a rechallenge is not permitted. (Chap. 23)

109. Answer: D

Lead poisoning is associated with cortical thinning of the prefrontal cortex, a phenomenon also associated with ADHD. (Chap. 11)

110. Answer: B

Desipramine has been associated with an increased risk of cardiotoxicity in prepubertal children. (Chap. 46)

111. Answer: C

Combining monoamine oxidase inhibitors with serotonergic agents can result in serotonin syndrome, which can include adverse events such as delirium, hyperthermia, autonomic instability, neuromuscular excitability, potential coma, and death. (Chap. 21)

112. Answer: D

Good specificity means the instrument will NOT detect a case when the person does NOT have the disorder and avoids false-positives. (Chap. 28)

113. Answer: A

Bulimia nervosa is categorized into purging and non-purging subtypes. (Chap. 40)

114. Answer: D

Manufacturers can advertise that their products can influence the structure or function of the body, provided they have substantiating evidence on file. They cannot claim that they prevent, cure, treat, or diagnose disease. (Chap. 25)

115. Answer: D

Naltrexone is an opiate antagonist that is used to reduce alcohol craving. Nalmefene, an opiate receptor antagonist, is another anti-craving agent being studied to treat alcohol addiction. (Chap. 41)

116. Answer: B

PECO is a mnemonic to remember the following in a clinical search query: the population of interest, exposure to active treatment, the control or comparison condition, and the desired outcome. (Chap. 29)

117. Answer: A

Nortriptyline and desipramine are tricyclic antidepressants that have been studied in ADHD. Reports of sudden unexplained death in four children with ADHD treated with desipramine engendered concerns about the safety of TCA use in children, although the causal link between TCAs and these deaths remains uncertain. (Chap. 31)

118. Answer: A

Pregnancy, hypothyroidism, and renal failure can be ruled out by obtaining human chorionic gonadotropin (hCG), thyroid-stimulating hormone (TSH), and creatinine levels, respectively. (Chap. 23)

119. Answer: A

Benzodiazepines are rapidly distributed to the brain once they enter the circulatory system and the rate-limiting step is absorption; anything that delays gastric emptying (e.g., co-administration of anticholinergic drugs) will delay the onset of action. (Chap. 24)

120. Answer: B

Atracurium and mivacurium are muscle relaxants that are used in ECT, but not as commonly as succinylcholine. (Chap. 26)

121. Answer: C

St. John's wort cannot generally be recommended in preference to selective serotonin reuptake inhibitors (SSRIs) for the treatment of depression in youths, given the lack of randomized controlled trials in children. The adult dosage of St. John's wort is 300 mg three times daily; in youths, clinicians have started at 150 mg three times daily, with an increase to 300 mg three times daily if it is well tolerated and there is no improvement. As with antidepressants, there is a 2- to 3-week lag of onset. (Chap. 25)

122. Answer: B

The relative potency of antipsychotics in increasing prolactin, from strongest to lowest, is as follows: paliperidone ≥ risperidone > haloperidol > olanzapine > ziprasidone > quetiapine > clozapine > aripiprazole. (Chap. 23)

123. Answer: C

Clomipramine can be used in OCD and has noradrenergic activity; studies have shown it can be helpful in ADHD. An SSRI and stimulant combination might be your first approach, however. An SSRI with bupropion can also be considered. (Chap. 35)

124. Answer: B

Treatment non-adherence in the context of the struggle for autonomy is not unusual. (Chap. 47)

125. Answer: B

Type II error or beta error is failing to reject the null hypothesis. That is, saying there is no difference in treatment arms when in fact there is. (Chap. 50)

126. Answer: A

Children have more efficient renal elimination. For example, children may eliminate lithium more rapidly than adults. (Chap. 3)

127. Answer: B

Youths with bipolar disorder take longer to recover when the initial mood episode is depression. (Chap. 33)

128. Answer: C

Treatment for ADHD may delay the onset of substance use and may be protective in adolescence itself, but overall, treatment has no impact on eventual substance use in adulthood. (Chap. 41)

129. Answer: D

Phase III trials are definitive trials for providing adequate evidence of efficacy for the claimed indications. (Chap. 51)

130. Answer: B

First-degree atrioventricular block is an example of a conduction delay. An ECG is recommended as a baseline study and, by some, once a therapeutic level has been attained. (Chap. 22)

131. Answer: A

Prenatal SSRI exposure with or without benzodiazepines for the treatment of maternal depression was associated with a reduced newborn behavioral response to pain induced by the PKU heel lance. (Chap. 44)

132. Answer: A and C

A seizure is the most serious potential side effect of TMS but is not the most common. (Chap. 26)

133. Answer: D

Carbamazepine was introduced in 1968 for the treatment of seizures and is structurally similar to imipramine. (Chap. 22)

134. Answer: A

The rate of children and adolescents receiving depression treatment is approximately 1 per 100 persons. Approximately half of those who receive treatment have received an antidepressant medication. (Chap. 49)

135. Answer: B

Olanzapine and risperidone are the best-studied antipsychotics in adult delirium. (Chap. 43)

136. Answer: B

Glucocorticoids provide inputs at the pituitary, hypothalamus, and other central sites involved in regulating the stress response. (Chap. 8)

137. Answer: B

Polycystic ovarian syndrome (PCOS) is an endocrine disorder resulting in ovulatory dysfunction and hyperandrogenism. There are increasing concerns about the possible association between valproate treatment in females and PCOS. (Chap. 22)

138. Answer: B

Ghrelin provides afferent signaling to the brain for the maintenance of body energy homeostasis. (Chap. 16)

139. Answer: B

Unconscious determinants were not assessed. Progress in school and the state of important relationships are important indicators of patient functionality. (Chap. 30)

140. Answer: B

Since co-administration of benzodiazepines with SSRIs during pregnancy may increase the risk of cardiac defects, it is important to limit their prescription during cardiogenesis. (Chap. 44)

141. Answer: B

Both duloxetine and venlafaxine are serotonin/norepinephrine reuptake inhibitors; however, at higher doses, both medications have more prominent noradrenergic reuptake inhibition. (Chap. 21)

142. Answer: B

Another anxiety disorder, substance use, and disruptive disorder are the most common disorders that co-occur with trauma. (Chap. 39)

143. Answer: A

Paroxetine has the highest risk ratio for suicidality among the SSRIs; however, venlafaxine, a serotonin norepinephrine reuptake inhibitor (SNRI), has a higher risk ratio. (Chap. 20)

144. Answer: B

Benzodiazepines may help with insomnia. There are no child studies, and adult studies of PTSD indicate that benzodiazepines have little effect on the core symptoms of re-experiencing, avoidance, and numbing. (Chap. 39)

145. Answer: E

Documenting informed consent is an important matter but is not related to the informed consent process. (Chap. 52)

146. Answer: B

Skin conductance reflects sympathetic nervous system activity. (Chap. 15)

147. Answer: C

Aggression is considered maladaptive if it is excessively impulsive or deliberately planned, unwarranted, and avoidable. (Chap. 47)

148. Answer: B

The AIMS examines side effects related to antipsychotic use and is limited to extrapyramidal side effects. (Chap. 18)

149. Answer: C

This has been reported in the literature at the case level. Resumption of growth and maturation after discontinuation is reported. The child may not recognize symptoms of this adverse effect and so may not report it. (Chap. 48)

150. Answer: C

ADHD is a clinical diagnosis. Neuropsychological testing can help in complicated cases or to determine cognitive functioning and learning disorders. Such testing is not sensitive to ADHD per se. (Chap. 31)

151. Answer: D

Prescriptions of antipsychotic agents increased 5- to 20-fold between 1996 and 2001 to rates of 0.8 to 5.5 per 1000 children. (Chap. 45)

152. Answer: A

Each option might be relevant for a given case, but of the options listed increased bleeding is the most concerning one to consider in patients with coagulopathies and thrombocytopenia. In patients who develop abnormal bleeding after starting SSRIs, possible underlying predisposing factors should be considered and evaluated. (Chap. 43)

153. Answer: D

The risk of children under 16 years developing a rash on lamotrigine treatment is 3 times greater than the risk for adults. (Chap. 22)

154. Answer: C

The mortality associated with ECT is approximately the same as that for anesthesia alone. (Chap. 26)

155. Answer: A

Benzodiazepines work throughout the CNS, but their action upon limbic and cortical areas is responsible for the anxiolytic effects. (Chap. 24)

156. Answer: B

There are also data from family studies on the associations between childhood GAD and adult major depression. (Chap. 10)

157. Answer: A

Children with autism spectrum disorders, in contrast with typically developing children, initially have greater amygdala volumes between the ages of 7.5 and 12.5 years but fail to progress with age-related volumetric increase. (Chap. 14)

158. Answer: D

Most pharmacological trials are aimed at testing the null hypothesis, namely that treatment and control have equal effect; if they do not have equal effect, the null hypothesis is rejected and treatment is considered superior. If comparing the treatment to an established treatment, one is not testing the null hypothesis directly (since the null hypothesis has already been rejected for the established treatment) but instead "non-inferiority." If there is no inferiority of treatment, within acceptable limits, the treatment is considered efficacious. (An example is testing treatment for ADHD against stimulant treatment.) (Chap. 50)

159. Answer: A

By definition, adverse events are symptoms that occur after or worsen after the start of treatment. This simple definition mandates a review of pre-existing function. Without this crucial step, the increased insomnia and limited appetite commonly identified in children with ADHD even prior to treatment, for example, has the potential to be spuriously attributed to the initiation of pharmacotherapy. (Chap. 27)

160. Answer: C

Tight binding to the CYP docking site and its destruction is mechanism-based in inhibition. (Chap. 4)

161. Answer: E

Cognitive side effects include impairment of working memory and verbal fluency. Rarely, hyperthermia has been reported in pediatric epilepsy patients treated with topiramate. There are case reports of potentially life-threatening, severe hyperthermia when used in combination with olanzapine. (Chap. 22)

162. Answer: B

The bell-and-pad method works best for enuresis; however, parasomnias or excessive deep sleep can confound the success of such alarm systems for nocturnal enuresis. (Chap. 48)

163. Answer: C

According to experts, SSRI medication should be considered after 4 to 6 weeks of CBT for OCD if there is a poor response to CBT alone. (Chap. 29)

164. Answer: D

33% of children diagnosed with separation anxiety disorder will manifest symptoms of at least one psychiatric disorder in adulthood. (Chap. 34)

165. Answer: A

Guanfacine and clonidine are alpha-2 agonists. (Chap. 19)

166. Answer: C

Autism is more common in males than females by a ratio of 4:1. (Chap. 38)

167. Answer: C

Pharmaceutical sponsors could gain an additional 6 months of market exclusivity (freedom from generic competition) either for new drugs (i.e., not yet approved) or for drugs already approved and marketed if they conducted pediatric studies. Importantly, the new law did not require that the study results be positive to support the additional exclusivity. (Chap. 51)

168. Answer: D

Mood symptoms respond well to ECT. AACAP guidelines recommend consideration of ECT in children who suffer from a severe psychiatric disorder, who are resistant to conventional treatment, and whose safety is compromised in waiting for a response from such treatment. (Chap. 26)

169. Answer: B

FDA approval of bupropion was delayed while the risk of seizures and other concerns were evaluated. (Chap. 21)

170. Answer: A

Prescription (hydroxyzine) and OTC (diphenhydramine) antihistamines are the most commonly prescribed or recommended sedatives in pediatric practice. (Chap. 46)

171. Answer: A

Melatonin may also improve total sleep time, but it has little effect on the number of middle-of-the-night awakenings. (Chap. 42)

172. Answer: C

Long-term controlled studies versus placebo or alternative non-drug treatment would be the only suitable way to address long-term medication effects on subtle aspects of human behavior, but may not be practicable. The other answer options may be suitable for discrete, more obvious effects. (Chap. 51)

173. Answer: C

Parental depression, social anxiety, older age, and severity of symptoms have all been associated with decreased response. (Chap. 34)

174–178. Answers

174-B; 175-A; 176-C, A; 177-C; 178-D.

These are FDA-labeled indications. Physicians may use medications off-label. (Chap. 51)

179. Answer: D

Olanzapine has been shown to improve BMI and to improve depression, aggression, and obsessions-compulsions, although the data remain limited. (Chap. 40)

180. Answer: D

The extent to which physicians consult with one another is unlikely to add meaningful information to current, basic pharmacoepidemiological studies. (Chap. 49)

181. Answer: C

In this randomized study of 167 girls, inpatient treatment predicted a poor prognosis and patients receiving specialized outpatient care had no better outcomes than patients treated in general mental health clinics. However, there was a considerable dropout rate in the study. (Chap. 40)

182. Answer: B

64 outpatients, mean age late 20s, showed reduced body weight and had less drive for thinness, body dissatisfaction, and anxiety on topiramate. Given topiramate's effect on cognition, however, it must be used judiciously. (Chap. 40)

183. Answer: C

Depression is the most frequent comorbidity in both childhood and adult-onset schizophrenia. (Chap. 13)

184. Answer: C

50% of OCD cases are familial. Early stressful events have been associated with the onset of pediatric OCD. (Chap. 11)

185. Answer: A and C

Executive functioning and verbal IQ were inversely associated with physical violence; however, executive functioning and verbal IQ were positively related to a high frequency of theft during childhood to early adulthood. (Chap. 15)

186. Answer: C

SSRIs work primarily through presynaptic inhibition of serotonin reuptake. (Chap. 20)

187. Answer: B

Several trials have compared a second-generation antidepressant with placebo, including fluoxetine, fluvoxamine, sertraline, citalopram, escitalopram, and the SNRI atomoxetine. SSRIs have had a significant advantage over placebo in reducing binge attacks and a modest effect on weight reduction in adults. Adolescents were not part of the trials. (Chap. 40)

188. Answer: B

The lowest prevalence of less than 1% is found in Germany, the United Kingdom, France, Norway, and Puerto Rico (a commonwealth of the United States); there is a moderate prevalence (1–3%) in Australia, Canada, Netherlands,

Israel, and Iceland and a relatively higher prevalence (>3%) in the United States. (Chap. 54)

189. Answer: D

Only 20% of CNS monoamine oxidase is MAO-A; the rest is MAO-B. (Chap. 21)

190. Answer: A

The children's version of the Yale-Brown Obsessive Compulsive Scale (CY-BOCS) is the gold standard for assessment and monitoring of response to treatment. It consists of 10 items with a 0-to-4 scale. (Chap. 35)

191. Answer: B

The maximum one-time dose for bupropion is 150 mg for the immediate-release formulation, 200 mg for the SR formulation, and 400 mg for the XR formulation. (Chap. 21)

192. Answer: B

Carbamazepine decreases lithium clearance and increases the risk of lithium toxicity. (Chap. 22)

193. Answer: B

The child must also meet four additional criterion symptoms for the diagnosis of MDD. (Chap. 32)

194. Answer: A

The face validity of a test refers to whether the instrument appears to measure what it sets out to measure; it is qualitative in nature. (Chap. 28)

195. Answer: B

The FDA has regulatory oversight over drugs, biological treatments, and medical devices. The FDA has the authority to sanction investigators, institutional review boards, and sponsoring institutions. (Chap. 52)

196–198. Answers
196-A, C, E; 197-B, G, H; 198-D, F. (Chap. 17)

199. Answer: B

A conflict of interest occurs when there is a risk that patient care or patient welfare will be compromised by a secondary interest. (Chap. 52)

200. Answer: A

Pregabalin reduces excitatory neurotransmitters, including glutamate, norepinephrine, and substance P. (Chap. 24)

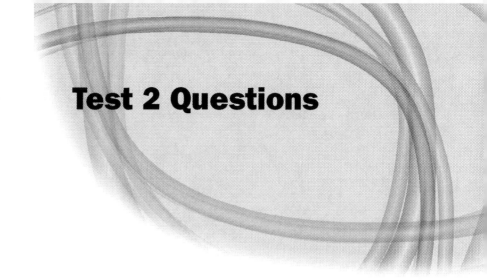

Test 2 Questions

1. What did a multi-site placebo-controlled trial of methylphenidate in children with attention-deficit/hyperactivity disorder (ADHD) find with regard to tics?

   A. The proportion of children reporting increased tics was greatest in the placebo group

   B. The proportion of children reporting increased tics was greatest in the methylphenidate group

   C. The proportion of children reporting decreased tics was greatest in the methylphenidate group

   D. The proportion of children reporting increased tics was the same in the methylphenidate and placebo groups

2. For the diagnosis of specific phobia prior to age 18, symptoms must be present for how long?

   A. 6 months

   B. 4 months

   C. 2 months

   D. 1 month

3. What proportion of youths in juvenile justice detention centers have an undiagnosed or undertreated psychiatric disorder?

   A. 15% or less

   B. 25%

   C. 45%

   D. 65% or more

4. Prolonged seizures (defined as longer than 150 seconds) in the course of electroconvulsive therapy (ECT) are important to identify because of their association with which complications?

   A. Greater postictal confusion

   B. Amnesia

   C. Cardiovascular complications

   D. All of the above

5. Children suffering from major depressive disorder (MDD) have a decreased occurrence of all the following symptoms compared with adolescents and adults EXCEPT:

   A. Melancholic symptoms

   B. Delusions

   C. Anhedonia

   D. Suicide attempts

6. Two recent large multi-site trials of children with autism treated for serious repetitive behaviors with citalopram or fluoxetine indicated:

   A. Much improvement in repetitive behaviors

   B. Moderate improvement in repetitive behaviors

   C. Mild improvement in repetitive behaviors

   D. Negative results

7. Which of the following is a must before starting pimozide?

   A. Complete blood count

   B. Electrocardiogram

   C. Liver enzymes

   D. No baseline studies are needed

8. Which of the following brain regions regulates attention?

   A. Inferior temporal cortex

   B. Posterior parietal association cortex

   C. Prefrontal cortex

   D. Basal ganglia

9. Studies aimed at examining preliminary evidence for safety and efficacy of medications are called:

   A. Phase 0 trials

   B. Phase I trials

   C. Phase II trials

   D. Phase III trials

   E. Phase IV trials

10. The weighted effect size for antidepressants in the treatment of pediatric aggression is small. The effect size is closest to:

    A. 0.3

    B. 0.5

    C. 0.8

    D. 1.2

11. All of the following statements are true EXCEPT:

    A. Women have lower WBC and ANC counts than men

    B. A subgroup of patients of African descent has habitually low white counts in the absence of any infections

    C. Benign ethnic neutropenia can be found in persons of African and Middle Eastern descent

    D. People of African descent have lower WBC and ANC counts than those of African-American descent

12. Which of the following anxiety disorders is the only one classified as a disorder first diagnosed in childhood?

    A. Generalized anxiety disorder

    B. Social phobia

    C. Separation anxiety disorder

    D. Anxiety, not otherwise specified

13. <u>Peak</u> serum concentrations of lithium are typically observed how long after each dose?

    A. 1 to 3 hours

    B. 2 to 4 hours

    C. 8 to 12 hours

    D. 14 to 18 hours

14. By late adolescence, what percentage of youths have met the criteria for major depressive disorder?

    A. 2%

    B. 5%

    C. 10%

    D. 25%

15. What is the dominant subclass of antidepressant in the industrialized world?

    A. Serotonin reuptake inhibitor

    B. Serotonin norepinephrine reuptake inhibitor

    C. Tricyclic

    D. Lithium

16. What is the best method to track weight changes when prescribing antipsychotics to children?

    A. Measure waist circumference

    B. Measure weight with shoes off

    C. BMI z-scores

    D. Absolute BMI

17. Which of the following brain structures plays a crucial role in body weight regulation?

    A. Hippocampus

    B. Amygdala

    C. Hypothalamus

    D. Dorsolateral prefrontal cortex

18. What term describes the elimination of a constant fraction of a drug independent of the amount circulating in the bloodstream?

    A. Zero-order kinetics

    B. First-order kinetics

    C. Non-linear kinetics

    D. Michaelis-Menten kinetics

19. Which of the following is the fast-acting postsynaptic receptor?

    A. Ionotropic receptor

    B. G-protein-coupled receptor

    C. Autoreceptor

    D. Heteroreceptor

20. The process of natural neuronal cell death carried out by a program encoded within the genome and starting with shrinkage and breakage of the chromatin in the nucleus is called:

    A. Migration

    B. Arborization

    C. Apoptosis

    D. Neurogenesis

21. Evidence from recent studies supports a model of the drug addiction process in which the acute and early effects are dopaminergic and the longer-term persisting vulnerability for relapse is:

    A. Dopaminergic

    B. Glutamatergic

    C. Serotonergic

    D. Noradrenergic

22. Which of the following appropriately describes pilot studies?

    A. The use of placebo may produce ambiguous or misleading results due to the small sample size

    B. If the clinical effect of a drug is meaningful but not large, a pilot study may not show a difference between groups

    C. If the effect of a drug is reported as large compared to placebo in a relatively small trial, this may suggest active treatment is superior to placebo

    D. All of the above

23. Which of the following major brain dopamine systems have been implicated in aggressive behaviors in animal studies?

    A. Nigrostriatal

    B. Mesolimbic

    C. Mesocortical

    D. All of the above

24. All the following have been adverse events associated with selective serotonin reuptake inhibitor (SSRI) treatment in children EXCEPT:

    A. Nausea and vomiting

    B. Restlessness

    C. Low energy

    D. Anhedonia

    E. Suicidal thinking

25. What is the lifetime prevalence of obsessive-compulsive disorder (OCD)?

    A. 0.5%

    B. 2% to 3%

    C. 8%

    D. 11%

    E. 15%

26. Behavioral disinhibition, which may occur in children given a benzodiazepine, may be overcome by:

    A. Providing a distracting, stimulating environment

    B. Adding diphenhydramine

    C. Increasing the dose

    D. Adding benztropine

27. What is the usual starting dose of clonidine for school-age children with Tourette's disorder?

    A. 0.025 mg QHS

    B. 0.05 mg QHS

    C. 0.1 mg QHS

    D. 1 mg QHS

28. What is the best definition of a tic?

    A. Sudden, rapid motor movement with associated vocal utterances

    B. Sudden, repetitive movement, gesture, or utterance that typically mimics some fragment of normal behavior

    C. Sudden, rapid vocal utterance with associated motor movements

    D. Sudden repetitive movement, gesture, or utterance that is a typical behavior

29. Why should lithium blood levels be monitored after labor and delivery?

    A. To manage potential postpartum mood disorder

    B. To reduce the risk of Ebstein's anomaly

    C. To account for rapid fluid shifts after parturition

    D. A and B

30. In which of the following disorders did ondansetron perform better than placebo in a small controlled trial?

    A. Schizophrenia

    B. Generalized anxiety

    C. Bulimia nervosa

    D. Intermittent explosive disorder

31. All the following conditions are considered high risk for undergoing electroconvulsive therapy (ECT) EXCEPT:

    A. Elevated intracranial pressure

    B. Type II diabetes

    C. Significant cardiac arrhythmia

    D. Severe valvular disease

32. Which of the following represents a pain syndrome that is usually localized to the distal upper or lower extremities, has sensory changes (such as pain to non-noxious stimuli) and autonomic changes (such as edema, abnormal color), and usually occurs after an inciting trauma?

    A. Complex regional pain syndrome

    B. Somatization disorder

    C. Somatoform disorder, not otherwise specified

    D. Pain disorder

33. In 1993, the American Academy of Pediatrics recommended against the use of chloral hydrate in children except for short-term sedation because of which prominent side effect?

    A. Cardiotoxicity

    B. Hepatotoxicity

    C. Acute renal failure

    D. Delirium

34. What percentage range of children with nighttime incontinence have a reversed (or decreased) arginine vasopressin (AVP) secretion with sleep?

    A. 1% to 2%

    B. 5% to 10%

    C. 15% to 25%

    D. 30% to 50%

35. Which of the following selective serotonin reuptake inhibitors (SSRIs) is least likely to have drug interaction effects?

    A. Paroxetine

    B. Fluoxetine

    C. Escitalopram

    D. Fluvoxamine

36. One reason tricyclic antidepressants are less widely used than other antidepressants is:

    A. The prolongation of the QTc interval

    B. The risk of hypertensive crisis after eating tyramine-rich foods

    C. The increased risk of metabolic adverse events

    D. The risk of seizures

37. A recent study of a population-based birth cohort of preschool-age children (N = 1950) whose developmental trajectories of physical aggression were assessed between the ages of 17 and 41 months found that frequent physical aggression was related specifically to which neurocognitive trait?

    A. Expressive language deficits

    B. Receptive language deficits

    C. Fine motor skills deficits

    D. Gross motor skills deficits

38. Which are the four bioethical principles that are often referred to in the current practice of medicine?

    A. Autonomy, beneficence, nonmaleficence, and patience

    B. Autonomy, beneficence, nonmaleficence, and justice

    C. Autonomy, munificence, nonmaleficence, and justice

    D. Autonomy, beneficence, non-munificence, and justice

39. When are adolescents with depression more likely to have elevated cortisol output?

    A. In the early morning prior to awakening

    B. Prior to sleep onset

    C. In the late afternoon

    D. In the middle of the night

40. **What is a parallel group design in a clinical trial?**

    A. Subjects are assigned randomly to one treatment of two or more alternatives

    B. Subjects are assigned randomly to treatment

    C. Subjects are given sequentially and in random order all the treatments that are being tested

    D. Subjects are assigned randomly to active treatment

41. **Psychopathy scores correlated with which of the following psychiatric diagnoses?**

    A. Histrionic personality disorder

    B. Borderline personality disorder

    C. Antisocial personality disorder

    D. All of the above

42. **Monoamine oxidase-A (MAO-A) preferentially deaminates which of the following biogenic amines?**

    A. Epinephrine

    B. Norepinephrine

    C. Serotonin

    D. All of the above

For questions 43–46, please list the corresponding finding

43. **Rett's disorder**

44. **Fragile X**

45. **Angelman**

46. **Prader-Willi**

    A. Imprinting, chromosome 15

    B. Trinucleotide expansion and methylation

    C. Methyl-CpG-binding protein 2 (MECP2) mutation

47. **What is the estimated lifetime prevalence of bipolar disorder in adults?**

    A. 1%

    B. 2%

    C. 4%

    D. 8%

48. **Which of the following tricyclic antidepressants was the first to be introduced for the treatment of depression?**

    A. Imipramine

    B. Amitriptyline

    C. Nortriptyline

    D. Desipramine

49. **Compared to adults, children have:**

    A. Less body water and relatively more adipose tissue

    B. An equivalent proportion of body water and adipose tissue

    C. Greater body water and relatively less adipose tissue

    D. None of the above

50. **When should prolactin levels be monitored in a patient on risperidone treatment?**

    A. Every 6 months

    B. Annually

    C. Only if there are symptoms of hyperprolactinemia

    D. Monitoring is not indicated

51. **Increased neurogenesis in rodents has been associated with which of the following?**

    A. Exposure to an enriched environment

    B. Learning tasks

    C. Running on an exercise wheel

    D. All of the above

For questions 52 to 56, match the drug with the correct FDA labeling for children and/or adolescents. A drug may have more than one correct corresponding answer option, or an answer option may correspond to more than one drug

52. **Aripiprazole**

53. **Chlorpromazine**

54. **Risperidone**

55. **Buspirone**

56. Sertraline

    A. Safety and efficacy not established for children with generalized anxiety disorder treated with adult doses

    B. Approved for the treatment of irritability associated with autistic disorder

    C. Approved for the treatment of schizophrenia

    D. Approved for the treatment of bipolar I disorder (may be for manic or mixed/manic)

    E. Approved for the treatment of severe behavioral problems in children and the short-term treatment of hyperactive children

    F. Approved for obsessive-compulsive disorder

57. In cases of true neuroleptic malignant syndrome (NMS), what are typical creatinine phosphokinase (CPK) levels?

    A. 10 or more

    B. 100 or more

    C. 300 or more

    D. 1000 or more

58. A recent epidemiological study recorded what percentage of psychopathology in children and adolescents with intellectual disability?

    A. 5% to 10%

    B. 11% to 18%

    C. 19% to 29%

    D. 31% to 41%

59. In Expert Consensus and Clinicians' Consensus surveys, which class of medications was rated most helpful in the treatment of patients with severe and persistent physical aggression and those who destroyed property?

    A. Beta-blockers

    B. Antidepressants

    C. Mood stabilizers

    D. Atypical antipsychotics

60. If an individual has obsessive-compulsive disorder (OCD), what is the risk of a first-degree relative having OCD?

    A. 8%

    B. 33%

    C. 66%

    D. 80%

    E. 100%

61. Which of the following is the most represented category of eating disorders clinically?

    A. Anorexia nervosa

    B. Bulimia nervosa

    C. Eating disorder, not otherwise specified

    D. Binge eating disorder

62. What precedes human testing of a new drug?

    A. Healthy volunteer trial

    B. Microdosing study

    C. Preclinical testing

    D. Phase 0 trial

63. Which of the following antipsychotics has a lower risk of weight gain?

    A. Olanzapine

    B. Risperidone

    C. Quetiapine

    D. Haloperidol

64. Which of the following agents has randomized controlled trials showing effectiveness in reducing anxiety symptoms in adults but has been linked with severe liver damage?

    A. Sertraline

    B. St. John's wort

    C. Paroxetine

    D. Kava

65. What is the main mechanism of action of alpha-2a adrenoreceptors?

    A. The receptor functions as an autoreceptor

    B. The receptor mediates the potent inhibitory effects of alpha-2 agonists on norepinephrine metabolism through the actions of the locus coeruleus

    C. Somatodendritic alpha-2a receptors suppress the excitability of locus coeruleus neurons

    D. Presynaptic alpha-2a receptors mediate the auto-inhibition of norepinephrine release

    E. All of the above

66. **Which alpha-2 receptor subtype is the predominant subtype found in the brain?**

    A.   Alpha-2a

    B.   Alpha-2b

    C.   Alpha-2c

    D.   Alpha-2d

67. **Which of the following best describes research experience with eating disorder, not otherwise specified, when compared to anorexia or bulimia?**

    A.   There is vast empiric support

    B.   There is a fear of gaining weight, amenorrhea, and very low body mass index

    C.   A patient engages in bulimic episodes but does not have other symptoms of bulimia

    D.   There is less severe eating disorder psychopathology, but higher or comparable rates of comorbid psychiatric disorders

68. **What study was a large multi-center trial comparing cognitive behavior therapy, fluoxetine, fluoxetine combined with cognitive behavioral therapy, and placebo?**

    A.   The Treatment for Adolescent Depression Study (TADS)

    B.   The Study of Adolescent Depression (SAD)

    C.   The Treatment for Major Depression in Adolescents Study (TMDAS)

    D.   The CBT and Fluoxetine Treatment Study (CoFTS)

69. **Which of the following statements best describes the psychosocial treatment of anorexia nervosa in children and adolescents?**

    A.   Individual interventions are most successful

    B.   Family-based interventions are most successful

    C.   Group interventions are most successful

    D.   Nutrition counseling has little value

70. **What is the approximate half-life of sertraline in children and adolescents?**

    A.   6 hours

    B.   24 hours

    C.   48 hours

    D.   72 hours

    E.   96 hours

71. **What is a unique feature of aripiprazole among antipsychotics?**

    A.   It is a potent dopamine D2 antagonist

    B.   It causes no weight gain

    C.   It may reduce prolactin levels below baseline

    D.   It is approved by the FDA only for bipolar disorder

72. **Across controlled trials, the ratio of suicidal ideation and behavior for older adults started on selective serotonin reuptake inhibitors compared to placebo is closest to:**

    A.   1:1

    B.   2:1

    C.   3:1

    D.   4:1

73. **Which of the following categories must be approved by the Secretary of the U.S. Department of Health and Human Services if research is to proceed?**

    A.   Research not involving more than minimal risk

    B.   Greater than minimal risk, but with the prospect of direct benefit to the subject

    C.   Greater than minimal risk with no prospect of direct benefit to the subject, but likely to yield generalizable knowledge about the individual's disorder or condition

    D.   Research that is not approvable in any of the above categories, but that presents an opportunity to understand, prevent, or alleviate a serious problem that affects the health and welfare of children

    E.   All of the above must be approved

74. **The N-methyl-ᴅ-aspartate receptor also binds which neurotransmitter besides NMDA?**

    A.   Serotonin

    B.   Glutamate

    C.   Kainic acid

    D.   Glycine

75. **In what stage of life do tics peak in severity?**

    A.   Early first decade

    B.   Late first decade

    C.   Early second decade

    D.   Late second decade

76. **What is the mechanism of action of buspirone?**

    A. Agonist of somatodendritic 5-HT1A autoreceptors

    B. Variable antagonist of postsynaptic 5-HT1A receptors

    C. Down-regulation of 5-HT2 receptors

    D. Increased turnover of dopamine and norepinephrine

    E. All of the above

77. **D-cycloserine is a partial agonist of which of the following receptors?**

    A. GABA

    B. NMDA

    C. NE

    D. DA

    E. 5-HT

78. **All the following are criteria articulated by the Institute of Medicine that may be useful in developing, evaluating, and enforcing institutional conflict of interest policies EXCEPT:**

    A. Transparency

    B. Proportionality

    C. Accountability

    D. Nepotism

    E. Fairness

79. **Which of the following brain regions synthesizes dopamine?**

    A. Substantia nigra pars reticulata

    B. Substantia nigra pars compacta

    C. Ventral striatum

    D. Locus coeruleus

80. **Bupropion's mechanism of action includes which of the following types of neurons?**

    A. Dopaminergic

    B. Anticholinergic

    C. Antihistaminergic

    D. Serotonergic

81. **When were the first clinical trials of stimulants for the treatment of children with symptoms equivalent to what is now called attention-deficit/hyperactivity disorder?**

    A. 1900s

    B. 1930s

    C. 1950s

    D. 1970s

82. **Which of the following is a key brain structure in inhibiting the stress response?**

    A. Corpus callosum

    B. Basal ganglia

    C. Hippocampus

    D. Cerebellum

83. **How many years typically elapse before bipolar disorder is diagnosed and treatment initiated?**

    A. 15 years

    B. 10 years

    C. 5 years

    D. 2 years

84. **In clinical trials, as the number of outcome measures increases, the likelihood of missing data increases. Patients with incomplete sets of outcome measures may have to be dropped from the analyses. Thus, whenever possible it is preferable to:**

    A. Identify outcome variables of equal weight that can inform on the primary outcome of interest

    B. Identify one outcome variable that can inform on the primary outcome of interest and eliminate all other outcome measures

    C. Identify one outcome variable that can inform on the primary outcome of interest and arrange the other outcome variables in hierarchical order

    D. Identify outcome variables of equal weight that can inform on many outcomes of interest at once

85. **Which of the following is a description of psycho-pharmacotherapy?**
    A. Single-provider integrated treatment
    B. Combined treatment
    C. Utilization of psychoactive medication and psychotherapy by a single provider
    D. All of the above

86. **Stimulating which area of the brain has the most evidence of efficacy when using transcranial magnetic stimulation (TMS) for adult depression?**
    A. Temporal cortex
    B. Dorsolateral prefrontal cortex
    C. Limbic cortex
    D. Parietal cortex

87. **The lead author of the study in the journal *The Lancet* originally suggesting a link between the MMR vaccine and autism (an idea that has since been refuted, and the article has been retracted) had which conflict of interest?**
    A. He had financial ties to device manufacturers
    B. He had financial ties to a legal group
    C. He had financial ties to drug manufacturers
    D. He had financial ties to herbal manufacturers

88. **Dopaminergic neurons from the ventral tegmental area (VTA) project primarily to which brain areas?**
    A. Caudate and putamen
    B. Nucleus accumbens and amygdala
    C. Frontal, cingulate, and entorhinal cortex
    D. B and C

89. **According to the National Institutes of Health policy, all research must:**
    A. Have a randomized design
    B. Obtain consent from both parent and child
    C. Provide active treatment
    D. Include members of racial/ethnic minority groups

90. **Which statement is accurate?**
    A. Plasma levels of stimulants cannot be obtained
    B. Plasma levels of stimulants correlate robustly with treatment effect
    C. The duration of plasma levels of stimulants does not correlate with clinical response
    D. Descending concentration of stimulants corresponds with treatment effect

91. **Which of the following is the most accurate statement regarding the controlled evidence for benzodiazepines in the treatment of pediatric anxiety?**
    A. Benzodiazepines have similar efficacy in children and adults
    B. Benzodiazepines are not efficacious in children
    C. Benzodiazepines are more efficacious in children than in adults
    D. Benzodiazepines are not prescribed off-label in children

92. **The rate of completed suicide in patients with epilepsy compared to the general population is:**
    A. The same
    B. 2 times the rate
    C. 5 times the rate
    D. 20 times the rate

93. **What is the time to peak plasma concentration for diphenhydramine?**
    A. 30 minutes
    B. 2 to 3 hours
    C. 8 hours
    D. 12 hours

94. **The extent of absorption is usually expressed as the fraction absorbed or:**
    A. Excretion
    B. Rate of absorption
    C. Distribution
    D. Bioavailability

95. A patient stable on risperidone treatment begins carbamazepine for seizures and begins experiencing auditory hallucinations and paranoia again. What could explain this relapse?

    A. Carbamazepine treatment can induce psychotic episodes

    B. Carbamazepine catalyzes the autoinduction of risperidone

    C. Carbamazepine is a CYP inhibitor of risperidone

    D. Carbamazepine decreases serum levels of many atypical antipsychotics

96. Which of the following agents has been observed to reduce substance abuse among youths with attention-deficit/hyperactivity disorder (ADHD) and mood disorders?

    A. Ondansetron

    B. Acamprosate

    C. Desipramine

    D. Bupropion

97. All of the following drugs bypass phase I metabolic reactions because they have a hydroxyl group EXCEPT:

    A. Lamotrigine

    B. Lorazepam

    C. Temazepam

    D. Clonazepam

    E. Oxazepam

98. Long-term lithium use in adults is associated with clinically significant reductions in:

    A. Glomerular filtration rate

    B. T4 levels

    C. Urinary concentration capacity

    D. Parathyroid hormone levels

    E. A and C

99. In children, hypertension is defined as repeated systolic and/or diastolic blood pressures greater than which percentile for age, sex, and height?

    A. 75th percentile

    B. 80th percentile

    C. 85th percentile

    D. 90th percentile

    E. 95th percentile

100. Problems with elimination typically account for what percentage of all pediatric urology visits?

    A. 5%

    B. 15%

    C. 25%

    D. 40%

101. Which of the following is an accurate statement about binge eating disorder in those over 18?

    A. Sibutramine is inferior to placebo in reducing binge attacks

    B. Sibutramine is equal to placebo in reducing binge attacks

    C. Sibutramine is superior to placebo in reducing binge attacks

    D. Sibutramine is superior to orlistat in reducing binge attacks

102. Several studies of stimulant treatment have shown all the following effects EXCEPT:

    A. Children with ADHD on stimulants have an increased ability to perceive peer communications

    B. Children with ADHD on stimulants have an increased self-perception

    C. Children with ADHD on stimulants have worsening peer bullying as both victims and instigators

    D. The behavior of other children when around children with ADHD is more positive when the children with ADHD are on stimulants

    E. Children with ADHD on stimulants have a better understanding of situational cues

103. Imipramine for enuresis has been found to have which direct effect on the bladder?

    A. Anticholinergic effect

    B. Serotonergic effect

    C. Adrenergic effect

    D. A and C

104. Pregabalin is generally studied for which category of disorders?

    A. Psychotic disorders

    B. Anxiety disorders

    C. Mood disorders

    D. Somatoform disorders

105. What is the age cutoff for the "early onset" specifier in the diagnosis of separation anxiety disorder?

    A. 6

    B. 8

    C. 10

    D. 12

106. The phenomenon of ultra-rapid cycling in bipolar disorder consists of mood disturbance that meets criteria for a manic, mixed, hypomanic, or major depressive episode in what frequency?

    A. Four or more cycles per year

    B. 5 to 364 cycles per year

    C. Greater than 365 cycles per year

    D. None of the above

107. In the setting of procedural pain and anxiety, which agent might be considered as an option?

    A. Haloperidol

    B. Risperidone

    C. Lorazepam

    D. Clonazepam

108. All the following have played a role in codifying ethical standards for health care EXCEPT:

    A. Nuremburg Code

    B. Helsinki Declaration of Human Rights

    C. National Research Act

    D. Belmont Report

    E. National Alliance on Mental Illness

109. The major environmental trigger for melatonin secretion by the pineal gland is:

    A. Increased light

    B. Decreased light

    C. Moonlight

    D. Sunshine

110. Long-term treatment of aggression in youths with risperidone has been studied and the effects of continued risperidone treatment versus placebo withdrawal were examined. What was the finding?

    A. Youths showed no statistically significant difference to symptom recurrence on placebo or risperidone treatment

    B. Youths on placebo had 37 days to symptom recurrence versus 119 days on risperidone

    C. Youths on placebo has 119 days to symptom recurrence versus 37 days on risperidone

    D. Youths on placebo had greater weight gain

111. The basic processes that control drug concentration in the body resulting from a given dose include:

    A. Absorption

    B. Distribution

    C. Metabolism

    D. Excretion

    E. All of the above

112. Which of the following is absorbed most rapidly?

    A. Lorazepam

    B. Diazepam

    C. Temazepam

    D. Clonazepam

113. *In utero* exposure to which of the following medications is associated with a higher incidence of neural tube defects?

    A. Lithium

    B. Valproic acid

    C. Carbamazepine

    D. B and C

114. Which of the following describes metabolite-intermediate-complex inhibition?

    A. Tight binding to CYP docking site without destruction of the site

    B. Reversible binding to CYP docking site

    C. Tight binding to CYP docking site with destruction of the site

    D. High-affinity binding to CYP docking site

115. Carbamazepine induces its own metabolism. This autoinduction is complete how long after achieving a fixed dose?

    A. 24 hours

    B. 3 to 5 days

    C. 8 to 10 days

    D. 1 to 2 weeks

    E. 3 to 5 weeks

116. What is the benefit of family involvement in treating substance-abusing youths?

    A. It increases the parents' access to substance use treatment for themselves

    B. Parents are better able to administer random urine drug screens

    C. Recovering siblings as models are the number-one protective factor for recovering youths

    D. Family involvement increases compliance and sustains abstinence

117. Which of the following barbiturates is the most commonly used anesthetic agent in electroconvulsive therapy (ECT)?

    A. Methohexital

    B. Pentobarbital

    C. Butabarbital

    D. Thiopental

118. In what decade did venlafaxine emerge as a treatment for depression?

    A. 1930s

    B. 1950s

    C. 1970s

    D. 1990s

119. Which of the following scales focuses on degrees of functioning in a patient?

    A. Clinical Global Impression-Improvement

    B. Clinical Global Impression-Severity

    C. Columbia Impairment Scale

    D. None of the above

120. One study examining the longitudinal nature of preschool psychopathology found that what percentage of children who met criteria during the preschool years continued to have the disorder 2 years later?

    A. 5%

    B. 20%

    C. 50%

    D. 90%

121. All the following medications increase valproate levels EXCEPT:

    A. Erythromycin

    B. Sertraline

    C. Cimetidine

    D. Risperidone

    E. Aspirin

Match the following posttraumatic stress disorder (PTSD) instruments to their description

122. The Child Posttraumatic Stress Reaction Index (CPTS-RI)

123. Child PTSD Symptom Scale (CPSS)

124. Traumatic Symptom Checklist for Children (TSCC)

    A. 26-item self-report measure that assesses the frequency of PTSD symptoms in children 8 to 16 years of age

    B. A self-report measure that assesses for PTSD symptoms in children 8 to 16 years of age and also has clinical scales that assess for anxiety, anger, depression, dissociation, and sexual concerns

    C. Semi-structured interview with 20 questions scored 0 to 4 administered to children 6 to 17 years of age

125. What type of mirtazapine dosing is associated with greater sedative effects?

    A. Lower doses

    B. Higher doses

    C. Both low and high doses

    D. Supratherapeutic doses

126. The Pediatric OCD Treatment Study (POTS) examined which of the following?

    A. Fluoxetine

    B. Citalopram

    C. Paroxetine

    D. Sertraline

127. A 14-year-old boy on chronic lithium treatment presents for a routine visit. Which of the following lab tests might you check once a year?

    A. TSH

    B. Serum electrolytes

    C. Serum calcium levels

    D. Creatinine

    E. ECG

128. Which of the following attributes of topiramate is FALSE?

    A. Moderately effective for weight loss

    B. An effective mood stabilizer

    C. May impair working memory and verbal fluency

    D. May cause severe hyperthermia in combination with olanzapine

129. There is an interest in the possible benefits of long-chain polyunsaturated fatty acid supplementation in childhood mental disorders. These include which two?

    A. Omega and omega-3

    B. Omega-1 and omega-3

    C. Omega-3 and omega-6

    D. Omega-12 and omega-24

130. Which of the following first gave the FDA authority to require pediatric studies for certain new and marketed drug and biological products?

    A. Pediatric Research Equity Act (PREA) of 2003

    B. Pediatric Use subsection under the Precautions section of labeling in 1979

    C. Food and Drug Administration Modernization Act (FDAMA) of 1997

    D. Food and Drug Administration Amendments Act (FDAAA) of 2007

    E. Pediatric Rule of 1998

131. Which of the following has demonstrated effectiveness for the treatment of obsessive-compulsive disorder (OCD)?

    A. Psychodynamic psychotherapy

    B. Exposure and response prevention

    C. Narrative therapy

    D. Interpersonal therapy

132. Which one of the following elements of an assessment informs prognosis and course of illness and delineates empirically validated treatments for that particular disorder?

    A. Treatment history

    B. Co-occurring disorders

    C. Family assessment

    D. Diagnosis

133. In treating attention-deficit/hyperactivity disorder (ADHD) comorbid with a tic disorder in a child who is medication-naïve, which of the following is ill advised?

    A. Methylphenidate

    B. Guanfacine

    C. Atomoxetine

    D. None of the above; all are reasonable options

134. What is the potential advantage of using clozapine in children who are in residential placement and who have bipolar disorder, intermittent explosive disorder, or posttraumatic stress disorder (PTSD)?

    A. The side-effect profile is better than most antipsychotics

    B. Sedation is less frequent

    C. It reduces polypharmacy of mood stabilizers and antidepressants

    D. Reduced sialorrhea

135. Which GABA receptors mediate fast synaptic inhibition via transmitter-gated chloride ion channels?

    A. $GABA_A$

    B. $GABA_B$

    C. $GABA_C$

    D. $GABA_A$ and $GABA_C$

    E. $GABA_A$ and $GABA_B$

136. Which of the following describes the increased risk of developing bipolar disorder for children with a parental history of bipolar disorder?

    A. Five-fold

    B. Three-fold

    C. Two-fold

    D. Slightly increased risk

137. Tryptophan, an herbal preparation used to promote sleep, has been associated with which safety concern?

    A. Eosinophilic myalgia syndrome

    B. Hepatotoxicity

    C. Acute renal failure

    D. Thrombocytopenia

    E. Leukocytosis

138. Benign rashes develop in 12% of adults on lamotrigine treatment and typically emerge within:

    A. The first few days of treatment

    B. The first 2 weeks of treatment

    C. The first 8 weeks of treatment

    D. The first 24 weeks of treatment

139. The adverse effect of akathisia has been reported with which of the following?

    A. Quetiapine

    B. Risperidone

    C. Ziprasidone

    D. All of the above

140. Which of the following medications had a FDA black box warning for the risk of liver failure and was later removed from the U.S. market?

    A. Trazodone

    B. Bupropion

    C. Nefazodone

    D. Nortriptyline

141. Which two disorders have been a focus of studies examining dopamine-related alleles?

    A. Major depressive disorder and attention-deficit/hyperactivity disorder

    B. Schizophrenia and attention-deficit/hyperactivity disorder

    C. Schizophrenia and posttraumatic stress disorder

    D. Generalized anxiety disorder and attention-deficit/hyperactivity disorder

142. An adult is considered to have decision-making capacity if he or she has information and understanding of each of the following elements EXCEPT:

    A. The physiological reason for and the etiology of the presenting condition

    B. The current medical situation/problem and prognosis

    C. The nature of the medical care being recommended by the treatment team

    D. The alternative courses of care

    E. The risks, benefits, and consequences for all alternatives, including those recommended and not recommended

143. Which of the following statements is accurate?

    A. There have been reported deaths by overdose of selective serotonin reuptake inhibitors (SSRIs) when they are ingested alone

    B. Deaths in overdose of SSRIs have occurred only in combination with other drugs

    C. SSRIs increase suicide completion

    D. Alcohol and SSRIs interact to prevent SSRI metabolism

144. Serotonin is produced from which amino acid?

    A. Lysine

    B. Tryptophan

    C. Tyrosine

    D. Glutamate

145. Which group writes the largest number of psychotropic prescriptions to children and adolescents?

    A. Nurse practitioners

    B. Pediatricians

    C. Psychiatrists

    D. Physician's assistants

146. If an oral contraceptive is abruptly discontinued, which of the following might occur for a patient taking lamotrigine?

    A. Acne

    B. Stevens-Johnson syndrome

    C. Weight gain

    D. Vivid dreams

147. If the specificity of a clinical screening instrument is 0.90, what is the false-positive rate?

    A. 2%

    B. 5%

    C. 10%

    D. 15%

148. Which of the following substances enhances GABA_A receptor functioning?

    A. Nicotine

    B. Cocaine

    C. Alcohol

    D. Opiates

149. The physician checks for hyperprolactinemia in a patient on an antipsychotic who complains of nipple discharge. The level is 190 ng/mL. Which strategy should the physician employ first?

    A. Obtain an MRI

    B. Reduce the dose

    C. Change the antipsychotic to haloperidol, if this has not been tried previously

    D. Prescribe bromocriptine

150. Coexisting psychiatric disorders among patients with childhood-onset schizophrenia are present in what percentage of patients?

    A. 10%

    B. 25%

    C. 50%

    D. 85%

151. After several weeks of treatment on a selective serotonin reuptake inhibitor (SSRI), which of the following happens?

    A. Alpha-adrenergic antagonism increases

    B. Cholinergic side effects emerge

    C. Serotonin receptors are methylated

    D. Serotonin receptors are down-regulated

152. A meta-analysis of randomized controlled trials in the pediatric population has shown which of the following agents to be superior in reducing obsessive-compulsive symptoms?

    A. Fluoxetine

    B. Paroxetine

    C. Fluvoxamine

    D. Clomipramine

153. The commercially available stimulants (methylphenidate, amphetamines) are structurally dissimilar but share a phenylethylamine backbone with catecholamines such as:

    A. Norepinephrine and dopamine

    B. GABA and glycine

    C. Serotonin and glutamate

    D. Dopamine and glycine

154. What is a fundamental finding of the initial, 14-month phase of the Multimodal Treatment Study for ADHD (MTA)?

    A. The core symptoms of ADHD respond equally to stimulants and behavioral intervention

    B. The core symptoms of ADHD respond to stimulants, and behavioral intervention does not add to this response

    C. Children with ADHD respond to stimulants and behavioral intervention is never needed

    D. Most children responded equally to placebo

155. The amount of individual CYPs may vary from person to person by up to what magnitude?

    A. 2-fold

    B. 5-fold

    C. 10-fold

    D. 50-fold

    E. 100-fold

156. National Ambulatory Medical Care Survey data from 1994–1995 and 2002–2003 show an increase in the diagnosis of bipolar disorder in children and adolescents, from 25 per 100,000 in 1994–1995 to _____ in 2002–2003

    A. 100 per 100,000

    B. 200 per 100,000

    C. 500 per 100,000

    D. 1000 per 100,000

157. In the clinically meaningful metric of effect size, a large magnitude of effect is represented by which of the following decimals?

    A. 0.2

    B. 0.4

    C. 0.6

    D. 0.8

158. What is the time period for organogenesis during gestation?

    A. The first 12 weeks

    B. The second trimester

    C. The third trimester

    D. The last 12 weeks

159. What are phase IV trials?

    A. Post-marketing studies to delineate additional information, including the drug's risks, benefits, and optimal use

    B. Initial studies to determine the metabolism and pharmacologic actions of drugs in humans and the side effects associated with increasing doses, and to gain early evidence of effectiveness; may include healthy participants and/or patients

    C. Controlled clinical studies conducted to evaluate the effectiveness of the drug for a particular indication(s) in patients with the disease or condition under study and to determine the common short-term side effects and risks

    D. Expanded controlled and uncontrolled trials after preliminary evidence suggesting effectiveness of the drug has been obtained; intended to gather additional information to evaluate the overall benefit/risk relationship of the drug and to provide an adequate basis for physician labeling

160. Which of the following explains why bupropion hydrochloride has been used to treat attention-deficit/hyperactivity disorder (ADHD)?

    A. It has noradrenergic and dopaminergic properties

    B. A part of the structure is related to the endogenous amphetamine-like substance phenylethylamine

    C. Controlled trials have demonstrated its effectiveness

    D. All of the above

161. Bipolar youths with substance use disorders, compared to those without one, have higher rates of all the following EXCEPT:

    A. Other comorbidities

    B. Medication compliance

    C. Treatment non-adherence

    D. Poorer overall functioning

162. A small companion study of risperidone by the Research Units on Pediatric Psychopharmacology (RUPP) Autism Network suggested that risperidone treatment for irritability in children and adolescents with autistic disorder required at least how many months of treatment to prevent relapse?

    A. 2 months

    B. 4 months

    C. 6 months

    D. 8 months

    E. 10 months

163. Which of the following medications, especially at higher doses, is associated with hypertension and requires blood pressure monitoring?

    A. Duloxetine

    B. Venlafaxine

    C. Bupropion

    D. Mirtazapine

164. Randomized controlled trials of antipsychotics in children and adolescents have evaluated all the following (with positive effects over placebo) EXCEPT:

    A. Pediatric bipolar mania

    B. Tic disorders

    C. Irritability associated with autistic disorder

    D. Disruptive disorders

    E. Posttraumatic stress disorder

165. Neural circuit loops are the biological substrates of habit formation and tics, connecting which areas of the brain?

    A. Limbic system with the cortex

    B. Hippocampus with the prefrontal cortex and thalamus

    C. Occipital cortex with the caudate nucleus and substantia nigra

    D. Basal ganglia with the cortex and thalamus

166. A meta-analysis found that electroconvulsive therapy (ECT) had what magnitude of effect size in 18 randomized controlled trials when comparing ECT with pharmacotherapy in 1144 patients?

    A. −0.2

    B. 0.2

    C. 0.4

    D. 0.8

167. Which acronym represents the study that examined the efficacy and tolerability of methylphenidate in stimulant-naïve preschoolers with moderate to severe ADHD?

    A. TADS

    B. POTS

    C. PATS

    D. MTA

168. Which of the following antipsychotics is contraindicated for use in the pediatric population due to QTc prolongation?

    A. Thioridazine

    B. Thiothixene

    C. Trifluoperazine

    D. Perphenazine

169. Most antidepressants, especially those with anticholinergic effects, suppress rapid eye movement (REM) activity and increase latency to REM sleep. If the medication is withdrawn abruptly, it may lead to which symptom?

    A. Dry mouth

    B. Delirium

    C. Increased nightmares

    D. Somnolence

    E. Constipation

170. If the lay public or other medical professionals are unaware of the prevalence of childhood mental illnesses, which of the following might result?

    A. Public policy changes

    B. School mental health screening

    C. Increased treatment

    D. The belief that medications are overprescribed

171. Zolpidem, zaleplon, and eszoplicone have which P450 enzyme in common for their metabolism?

    A. CYP2B6

    B. CYP2C19

    C. CYP1A2

    D. CYP3A4

172. Maternal depression and anxiety during pregnancy have been associated with an increased risk for developing:

    A. Preterm labor

    B. Pre-eclampsia

    C. Placental abruption

    D. Gestational diabetes

173. Gabapentin may sometimes cause which of the following symptoms when given to younger children?

    A. Post-herpetic neuralgia

    B. Partial seizures

    C. Behavioral disinhibition

    D. Toxic epidermal necrolysis

174. The Cannabis Youth Treatment Study, a multi-site randomized trial involving 600 adolescents, included all the following treatment approaches EXCEPT:

    A. Motivational enhancement therapy

    B. Interpersonal therapy

    C. Adolescent community reinforcement approach

    D. Multidimensional family therapy

175. The rate at which a non-twin sibling of a child with Tourette's disorder is affected is:

    A. 1%

    B. 5% to 10%

    C. 40% to 60%

    D. 60% or more

176. A 2-week drug-free interval is recommended in order to avoid serotonin syndrome when switching from a monoamine oxidase inhibitor (MAOI) to which antidepressant?

    A. Fluoxetine

    B. Venlafaxine

    C. Phenelzine

    D. All of the above

177. In medically ill patients who are agitated, what is the main concern for using antihistamines?

    A. They help induce sleep

    B. They have anticholinergic effects

    C. They frequently lead to pruritus

    D. They have a narrow therapeutic index

178. All of the following are the most frequent clinical manifestations of childhood insomnia, particularly in younger children, EXCEPT:

    A. Bedtime refusal or resistance

    B. Delayed sleep onset

    C. Early-morning awakening

    D. Prolonged night awakening

179. A drug reaction in which a child on sertraline develops a hyperserotonergic state after tramadol is added to treat pain is known as a:

    A. Pharmacogenetic reaction

    B. Pharmacodynamic reaction

    C. Pharmacokinetic reaction

    D. None of the above

180. Which of the following statements is true?

    A. Manufacturers of dietary supplements must register with the FDA

    B. Manufacturers of dietary supplements are regulated by the FDA

    C. Manufacturers of dietary supplements are responsible for ensuring that a dietary supplement is safe before marketing it

    D. Advertising by the dietary supplement industry is regulated by the FDA

181. Which psychiatric disorder is associated with the highest rate of suicide in adulthood?

    A. Bipolar disorder

    B. Schizophrenia

    C. Major depressive disorder

    D. Generalized anxiety disorder

182. Valproate is readily absorbed from the gastrointestinal system and reaches peak levels how many hours after each dose?

    A. 1 to 2

    B. 2 to 4

    C. 6 to 10

    D. 12 to 16

183. Which of the following is the primary plasma-binding protein in the body?

    A. Alpha-1-acid glycoprotein

    B. Albumin

    C. C-reactive protein

    D. Retinol binding protein

184. What is the dose range of clonidine for the treatment of attention-deficit/hyperactivity disorder (ADHD) in children?

    A. 10 to 30 mg

    B. 1 to 3 mg

    C. 0.1 to 0.3 mg

    D. 100 to 300 mg

185. Which of the following should be given routinely to patients with anorexia?

    A. Calcium and vitamin D

    B. Calcium and potassium

    C. Vitamin D and potassium

    D. Calcium and magnesium

186. What strategy can be used to reduce the peak level of a drug—and thus reduce side effects—without altering the total dose (i.e., the area under the curve) that is delivered?

    A. Split the dose over the day

    B. Administer without fatty food

    C. Deliver the dose intravenously when feasible

    D. All of the above

187. What percentage of patients who were noncompliant with lithium relapsed in an 18-month naturalistic prospective study of bipolar adolescents?

    A. 15%

    B. 30%

    C. 45%

    D. 90%

188. In 2004, the pharmaceutical industry in the United States spent roughly what portion of their overall sales on promotion and advertising?

    A. One-eighth

    B. One-fifth

    C. One-fourth

    D. One-third

189. All of the following areas of research could help understand prescribing patterns and medication practice in children and adolescents EXCEPT:

    A. Ethnic differences in medication use

    B. The licensing requirements of the Drug Enforcement Agency

    C. Availability of community resources

    D. The effect of managed care polices

    E. Physician and non-physician prescriber and parent attitudes towards medication use

190. Which of the following is the pulse width of the electrical stimulus used in modern electroconvulsive therapy (ECT)?

    A. 2 to 3 seconds

    B. 0.5 to 2 seconds

    C. 2 to 3 milliseconds

    D. 0.5 to 2 milliseconds

191. Established under the auspices of the FDA for review and monitoring of clinical drug trials, the composition of this group varies but typically includes clinicians familiar with the particular study population, a biostatistician, clinical pharmacologist, toxicologist, and often epidemiologist and bioethicist

    A. Institutional Review Board

    B. Center for Drug Evaluation and Research

    C. Data Monitoring Committee or Data Safety Monitoring Board

    D. The National Institutes of Health

192. Which of the following selective serotonin reuptake inhibitors (SSRIs) is FDA-approved for the treatment of adolescent depression?

    A. Fluoxetine

    B. Sertraline

    C. Escitalopram

    D. A and C

193. Which of the following statements is most accurate for clonidine prior to treatment or during treatment?

    A. A resting pulse of less than 60 beats per minute should prompt additional detailed evaluation or dose reduction

    B. A blood pressure measurement greater or lesser than 1 standard deviation from age- and gender-based means should prompt additional evaluation before treatment

    C. Orthostatic pulse or blood changes of greater than 5% should raise concern as to whether the dose should be decreased

    D. A, B, and C

    E. None of the above

194. **What is a reason children with posttraumatic stress disorder (PTSD) often show signs of attention-deficit/hyperactivity disorder (ADHD) and other disruptive disorders?**

    A. The diagnostic and statistical manual (DSM) criteria overlap

    B. Comorbidity is common in PTSD

    C. Brain areas involved in the stress response also modulate motor behavior

    D. Children with PTSD live in psychosocial circumstances that promote ADHD

195. **Which of the following best characterizes the clinical use of clonidine?**

    A. Was first used in the treatment of tics and later in the treatment of hypertension

    B. Was first used in the treatment of hypertension and later in the treatment of tics

    C. Was first used in the treatment of glaucoma and later in the treatment of tics

    E. Was first used in the treatment of nausea and later in the treatment of tics

196. **Which term describes the relevance of a screening instrument for the construct being measured rated by a panel of experts?**

    A. Face validity

    B. Content validity

    C. Positive predictive power

    D. Negative predictive power

197. **At what age does biological motion perception (the visual perception of a biological creature engaged in a recognizable activity) emerge in humans?**

    A. 3 years old

    B. 2 years old

    C. 2 months old

    D. 2 days old

198. **All the following are part of the DSM-IV criteria for obsessive-compulsive disorder EXCEPT:**

    A. Must cause subjective distress (suffering)

    B. Must be time-consuming (usually taking at least 1 hour a day)

    C. Compulsions must accompany obsessions

    D. Can cause functional impairment in one or more domains of life

199. **Which of the following attributes in children with an autism spectrum disorder is a strong predictor of eventual outcome?**

    A. Language skills

    B. Seizures

    C. IQ

    D. Adaptive skills

    E. A and D

200. **The Tourette's Syndrome Study Group found that:**

    A. Methylphenidate should be avoided in children with pre-existing tics

    B. Methylphenidate and clonidine were effective for ADHD

    C. Clonidine alone was as effective as methylphenidate alone

    D. Clonidine was not effective for ADHD

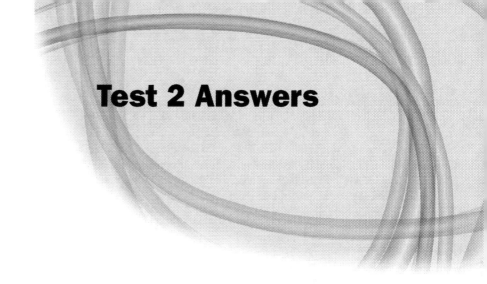

Test 2 Answers

1. Answer: D

In the Tourette's Syndrome Study Group, the proportion of children reporting a worsening of tics was 22% for the methylphenidate group and 20% for the placebo group, essentially the same statistically. Other studies have found otherwise; overall, the recent literature supports the use of stimulants in tics with risks and benefits weighed. (Chap. 31)

2. Answer: A

6 months. Typical onset of specific phobia occurs during childhood. (Chap. 10)

3. Answer: D

Approximately two-thirds or more of youths in juvenile detention centers have undiagnosed or undertreated psychiatric illness, with many meeting criteria for three or four diagnoses. Comorbid substance use is also a frequent finding. (Chap. 47)

4. Answer: D

Cardiovascular, as well as cerebral, complications are hypoxia-related risks associated with prolonged seizures during the course of ECT. (Chap. 26)

5. Answer: C

Anhedonia is found at rates comparable to adults. The differences in symptoms of MDD between children and adults can be attributed to the difference in developmental stages. (Chap. 32)

6. Answer: D

No effect with citalopram or fluoxetine was noted for repetitive behaviors in children with autism. (Chap. 42)

7. Answer: B

Pimozide increases the QT interval and an EKG should be obtained before initiation, during dose adjustment, at maintenance dose, and yearly thereafter. (Chap. 36)

8. Answer: C

The prefrontal cortex regulates attention, inhibits processing of irrelevant stimuli, and sustains and coordinates attention. (Chap. 11)

9. Answer: C

Studies that examine the preliminary evidence of safety and efficacy of medications are phase II trials; typically they have a sample size of 100 subjects or less. (Chap. 50)

10. Answer: A

0.3 corresponds to a small effect size, so this is the logical choice for the answer. (Chap. 47)

11. Answer: A

Men tend to have lower WBC and ANC values than women, not the other way around. As a result of the findings regarding WBCs in certain ethnic populations, adjustments to thresholds for neutropenia has been proposed. (Chap. 23)

12. Answer: C

Symptoms of separation anxiety disorder (SAD) must begin before age 18. SAD typically develops during middle childhood. (Chap. 10)

13. Answer: B

Peak serum concentrations of lithium are typically observed 2 to 4 hours after each dose. (Chap. 22)

14. Answer: D

Approximately 25% of youths have met criteria for major depressive disorder by late adolescence. (Chap. 9)

15. Answer: A

Serotonin reuptake inhibitors are the dominant subclass of antidepressants. (Chap. 54)

16.   Answer: C

BMI itself will not allow give sufficient data, since the implication of a given BMI varies across ages. The BMI z-score (standard deviation) is the most useful of the options listed. Age-adjusted BMI is also another method that is useful since BMI percentiles and z-scores have restricted tails at the upper and lower end. (Chap. 23)

17.   Answer: C

The hypothalamus has connections to the brain stem, midbrain, amygdala, hippocampus, and cortex, and if it is selectively lesioned or stimulated, predictable alterations in feeding behavior will occur. (Chap. 16)

18.   Answer: B

Answers A, C, and D are synonyms for one another. (Chap. 3)

19.   Answer: A

The class I, ionotropic receptors are the fast-acting receptors of the postsynaptic cell. (Chap. 2)

20.   Answer: C

During the early phase of central nervous system maturation, neurons are produced in excess and are later eliminated by apoptosis. (Chap. 1)

21.   Answer: B

Glutamatergic. Prolonged exposure to drugs appears to cause complex dysregulation of neural circuitry, which leads to long-term dependence even after the termination of drug use. (Chap. 17)

22.   Answer: D

Pilot studies have advantages and disadvantages that relate to sample size and its effect on results. (Chap. 50)

23.   Answer: D

All major brain dopamine systems appear to be involved in the rewarding or reinforcing aspects of aggression and/ or the initiation, execution, and termination of aggressive behavior patterns. (Chap. 15)

24.   Answer: D

Anhedonia is not considered a side effect of SSRI treatment. (Chap. 34)

25.   Answer: B

The lifetime prevalence of OCD is 2% to 3%. (Chap. 11)

26.   Answer: C

The phenomenon of behavioral disinhibition has not been well studied; however, disinhibition can generally be overcome by increasing the dose, since sedation increases as the dose escalates. (Chap. 24)

27.   Answer: B

The usual starting dose of clonidine is 0.05 mg in the evening. (Chap. 36)

28.   Answer: B

A tic is a sudden, repetitive movement, gesture, or utterance that typically mimics some fragment of normal behavior. (Chap. 12)

29.   Answer: C

Rapid fluid shifts occur in the maternal body after labor and delivery and can have a dramatic influence on lithium levels. (Chap. 44)

30.   Answer: C

Ondansetron, a 5-HT$_3$ antagonist, was self-administered before urges or, if there were no urges to eat, 30 minutes before food intake. Patients in the active drug group reported significantly reduced binging and purging. (Chap. 40)

31.   Answer: B

High-risk conditions for ECT also include unstable coronary syndrome, decompensated congestive cardiac failure, recent myocardial infarct, and stroke. There are no absolute contraindications for ECT, however. (Chap. 26)

32.   Answer: A

Complex regional pain syndrome type I (also called reflex sympathetic dystrophy [RSD]) has no definable nerve lesion. CRPS type II (or causalgia) has a definable nerve legion. Physical and occupational therapies along with cognitive behavioral therapy are agreed-upon treatments. The role of nerve blockade or neuropathic pain medications is less clear. (Chap. 43)

33.   Answer: B

Hepatotoxicity can be one of chloral hydrate's severe adverse effects. (Chap. 46)

34.   Answer: D

Humans typically secrete higher levels of AVP when asleep; however, 30 to 50% of children with nocturnal enuresis have a reversed (decreased) secretion of AVP while asleep resulting in increased urinary output. (Chap. 48)

35.   Answer: C

Sertraline and citalopram are also less likely to show drug interactions than fluoxetine, paroxetine, or fluvoxamine. (Chap. 32)

36. Answer: A

The effect on heart rate intervals such as QTc is the most severe adverse event for tricyclic antidepressants: they can be lethal in overdose by causing complete heart block or other fatal arrhythmias. (Chap. 21)

37. Answer: B

In this cohort of preschool children, frequent physical aggression was related specifically to receptive vocabulary deficits. (Chap. 15)

38. Answer: B

Autonomy, beneficence, nonmaleficence, and justice are the primary principles that guide care today. (Chap. 52)

39. Answer: B

Rather than having increased cortisol secretion throughout the day as depressed adults do, depressed adolescents are more likely to have elevated cortisol output close to the period of sleep onset, when the hypothalamic-pituitary-adrenal (HPA) axis is normally quiescent. (Chap. 9)

40. Answer: A

Most pharmacology trials are of parallel group design, where patients are assigned randomly to one treatment of two or more alternatives. (Chap. 50)

41. Answer: D

Psychopathy scores correlated with histrionic, borderline, and adult antisocial personality disorders. (Chap. 15)

42. Answer: D

Both MAO-A and MAO-B deaminate dopamine and tyramine; only MAO-A also deaminates the other amines. (Chap. 21)

43–46. Answers

43-C, 44-B, 45-A, 46-A.

The triplet repeat expansion in Fragile X syndrome is located on the long arm of the X chromosome on the FMR1 gene. In the case of Angelman there is a defect on maternal chromosome 15, and in Prader-Willi there is a defect on paternal chromosome 15. In Rett's disorder there is a mutation in the MECP2 gene. (Chap. 5)

47. Answer: C

The lifetime prevalence of bipolar disorder in adults is approximately 4%. (Chap. 33)

48. Answer: A

By the late 1950s, imipramine had gained worldwide recognition for the treatment of depression. Amitriptyline was the second tricyclic antidepressant to be developed. (Chap. 21)

49. Answer: C

Children have greater body water and less adipose tissue compared to adults. This difference can affect drug distribution and the kinetics of lipophilic drugs and metabolites. (Chap. 3)

50. Answer: C

Prolactin levels should be monitored only if there are symptoms suggestive of hyperprolactinemia. (Chap. 37)

51. Answer: D

Increase in neurogenesis is associated with an enriched environment, learning tasks, and exercise. Conversely, stress strongly decreases the proliferation of adult neuronal progenitor cells. (Chap. 1)

52–56. Answers

52-B, C, D; 53-C; 54-B, C, D; 55-A; 56-F.

These are FDA-labeled indications. Physicians may use medications off-label. (Chap. 51)

57. Answer: D

CPK levels are typically found to be 1000 or higher in cases of true NMS. (Chap. 23)

58. Answer: D

Several studies have reported that the prevalence of psychopathology is 3 to 6 times higher than the general population in people with intellectual disability. (Chap. 42)

59. Answer: D

Mood stabilizers were rated second in helpfulness in treating behaviors of physical aggression and destruction of property. (Chap. 42)

60. Answer: A

Although there is a large genetic component to OCD, for a given proband the risk of OCD in a first-degree relative is only 8% (compared to 2% in controls). (Chap. 11)

61. Answer: C

Although eating disorder, not otherwise specified, is the most clinically represented category, it is the least studied. (Chap. 16)

62. Answer: C

Preclinical testing is done with animals. (Chap. 51)

63. Answer: D

Haloperidol, aripiprazole, ziprasidone, and molindone have a lower risk of weight gain. (Molindone is not available in the U.S. market.) (Chap. 37)

64. Answer: D

Kava is effective for anxiety but has been linked to severe liver damage; as such it should be avoided in children, by people with liver problems, and in those taking drugs that can affect the liver. (Chap. 25)

65. Answer: E

Alpha-2a receptors are autoreceptors that mediate the inhibition of norepinephrine release through actions at the locus coeruleus. (Chap. 19)

66. Answer: A

Alpha-2a is the predominant alpha-2 subtype found in the brain, with large numbers in the locus coeruleus and other noradrenergic areas. Alpha-2d does not exist. (Chap. 19)

67. Answer: D

Eating disorder, NOS, has less severe eating disorder pathology but frequent comorbid psychiatric illness. (Chap. 40)

68. Answer: A

The TADS is the second largest psychopharmacology trial in children or adolescents after the Multimodal Treatment for ADHD Study (MTA). The fluoxetine vs. pill placebo arm showed that 61% responded to fluoxetine compared to 35% for placebo. The other options are fictitious. (Chap. 20)

69. Answer: B

Family-based interventions have the most evidence for success, regardless of design used. In contrast, for adult patients family work has generally been shown to be detrimental to treatment. (Chap. 40)

70. Answer: B

The half-life of sertraline is 26 hours in children and 27 hours in adolescents. (Chap. 20)

71. Answer: C

Aripiprazole, by virtue of its partial agonism at D2, may reduce prolactin levels below baseline. (Chap. 23)

72. Answer: A

For children, adolescents, and young adults the increased risk is 2:1. For older adults, there is no increased risk, or there may in fact be a decreased risk. (Chap. 51)

73. Answer: D

Research not approvable in the other listed categories, A–C in the answer options, must be approved by the Secretary of the U.S. Department of Health and Human Services after consultation with a panel of experts. (Chap. 52)

74. Answer: B

NMDA receptors primarily bind NMDA and glutamate. (Chap. 22)

75. Answer: C

Tics peak in severity in the early second decade of life and tend to decline by the end of the second decade of life. (Chap. 36)

76. Answer: E

Buspirone acts as an agonist of somatodendritic 5-HT$_{1A}$ autoreceptors, has variable antagonist effects on postsynaptic 5-HT$_{1A}$ receptors, down-regulates 5-HT$_2$ receptors, and increases dopamine and norepinephrine turnover. (Chap. 24)

77. Answer: B

NMDA is a subclass of glutamate receptor. (Chap. 38)

78. Answer: D

Proportionality, transparency, accountability, and fairness are the criteria the IOM proposes for conflict-of-interest policies. (Chap. 53)

79. Answer: B

The substantia nigra pars compacta synthesizes dopamine. (Chap. 11)

80. Answer: A

Bupropion's mechanism of action is not fully understood, but it appears to affect dopaminergic and noradrenergic mechanisms and has an absence of anticholinergic and antihistaminergic effects. (Chap. 21)

81. Answer: B

The first clinical trials were in the 1930s, with the role of stimulants well established by the 1970s. (Chap. 18)

82. Answer: C

The hippocampus, through direct and indirect inputs, inhibits corticotrophin-releasing hormone in the hypothalamus and reduces norepinephrine release from the locus coeruleus. (Chap. 8)

83. Answer: B

There is a 10% lower likelihood of recovery for each year of illness, which makes early recognition and treatment essential. (Chap. 33)

84. Answer: C

Missing data cannot always be estimated and may have to be dropped in the analysis. It is preferable to identify an outcome variable that can inform the primary outcome of interest and arrange the others in hierarchical order. The primary outcome variable should be sensitive to treatment effect and easily interpretable from a clinical perspective. (Chap. 50)

85. Answer: D

All answers are ways of describing psychopharmacotherapy, which has become less common in current psychiatric practice. (Chap. 30)

86. Answer: B

The optimal use of TMS has not been determined, but stimulating the dorsolateral prefrontal cortex is the approach that has the most evidence for efficacy. (Chap. 26)

87. Answer: B

Andrew Wakefield, the lead author of a study published in The Lancet that suggested a link between autism and the measles-mumps-rubella (MMR) vaccine, had not disclosed a highly relevant conflict of interest. In this case, the Legal Aid Board had commissioned him to determine—for a sizable fee—if evidence sufficed to support a legal action by parents of children allegedly harmed by the vaccine. Fear of the vaccine after publication led to a 20-fold increase in measles. (Chap. 53)

88. Answer: D

VTA neurons projecting to the nucleus accumbens and amygdala are called mesolimbic projections and those projecting to the frontal, cingulate, and entorhinal cortex are called mesocortical projections. (Chap. 2)

89. Answer: D

All research must include females and members of racial/ethnic minority groups unless a clear and compelling rationale is provided indicating that inclusion is inappropriate with respect to the health of the subjects or purpose of the research. The requirement for gender and ethnic inclusion can also be waived when prior research has definitely excluded the presence of clinically significant treatment effects among subgroups. (Chap. 50)

90. Answer: C

Duration of plasma levels has not been shown to correlate with response. An ascending concentration and slow, steady-state rising dopamine levels that mimic tonic firing are proposed to exert the therapeutic effect. (Chap. 18)

91. Answer: B

Benzodiazepines have not demonstrated efficacy in three placebo-controlled trials, although these studies had small sample sizes. (Chap. 34)

92. Answer: C

The rate of completed suicide in epilepsy patients is 5 times the rate in the general population. The rate is 25 times for those with temporal lobe epilepsy (partial complex seizures). (Chap. 43)

93. Answer: B

The time to peak concentration for diphenhydramine is 2 to 3 hours. (Chap. 24)

94. Answer: D

Bioavailability is synonymous with the extent of absorption. (Chap. 3)

95. Answer: D

Carbamazepine decreases the serum levels of many atypical antipsychotics. (Chap. 22)

96. Answer: D

Bupropion might be useful for substance-abusing youths with ADHD and/or mood disorders. (Chap. 41)

97. Answer: D

Lamotrigine, lorazepam, temazepam, and oxazepam bypass phase I reactions. (Chap. 4)

98. Answer: E

Long-term lithium use in adults is associated with clinically significant reductions in glomerular filtration rate and maximum urinary concentration capacity. (Chap. 22)

99. Answer: E

Hypertension is defined as repeated systolic and/or diastolic blood pressures at or above the 95th percentile for age, sex, and height. Pre-hypertension is defined as blood pressures at the 90th to 95th percentiles. Percentiles are available at http://www.nhlbi.nih.gov/health/prof/heart/hbp/hbp_ped.pdf. (Chap. 27)

100. Answer: D

Problems with elimination account for 40% of all pediatric urology visits. (Chap. 48)

101. Answer: C

Sibutramine, withdrawn from the US market, was superior to placebo in reducing binge eating attacks in patients 18 years of age and older who had binge eating disorder. (Chap. 40)

102. Answer: C

Children with ADHD on stimulants do better in a number of realms of social impairment; bullying is not worse. (Chap. 31)

103. Answer: D

Imipramine has an anticholinergic effect that increases bladder capacity and a noradrenergic effect that decreases detrusor muscle spasms and increases activity of the bladder neck and proximal urethra. (Chap. 42)

104. Answer: B

Pregabalin has an indication in the United States for neuropathic pain and fibromyalgia. Effectiveness has been demonstrated in social phobia and generalized anxiety disorder in adults. (Chap. 24)

105. Answer: A

If separation anxiety disorder occurs before age 6, the specifier "early onset" is assigned. (Chap. 34)

106. Answer: B

Pediatric bipolar disorder appears more complex than the adult disorder with the presence of short cycles embedded with a more prolonged episode that can include ultra-rapid or ultradian cycling. (Chap. 33)

107. Answer: C

Lorazepam can be useful for anxiety associated with procedural pain. It can be delivered PO or IV (or IM for other indications) without dose adjustment for a given route, making it easier to administer. (Chap. 43)

108. Answer: E

NAMI as an advocacy organization plays a role in ethics, but the other answer options have more directly set standards for ethics in research and care. The role of institutional review boards emerged with the National Research Act. The Belmont Report informed current ethical regulations. (Chap. 52)

109. Answer: B

Decreased light promotes melatonin secretion by the pineal gland. (Chap. 46)

110. Answer: B

Youths maintained on risperidone had a longer time to symptom recurrence. (Chap. 47)

111. Answer: E

Collectively, these processes are referred to as ADME, which describes the pharmacokinetics of a particular drug and its form of dosing. These four processes determine the duration of drug action. (Chap. 3)

112. Answer: B

Diazepam is absorbed at a rapid rate, leading to a fast onset of action. (Chap. 24)

113. Answer: D

The rate of neural tube defects in the general population is 0.038% to 0.096%. However, in utero exposure to either valproic acid or carbamazepine is associated with an 1% to 2% incidence of neural tube defects. (Chap. 44)

114. Answer: A

Tight binding to the CYP docking site without its destruction is metabolite-intermediate-complex inhibition. (Chap. 4)

115. Answer: E

Carbamazepine autoinduces its own metabolism, and this occurs after 3 to 5 weeks on a fixed dose. (Chap. 22)

116. Answer: D

Family involvement in substance-abusing youths increases compliance and sustains treatment. (Chap. 41)

117. Answer: A

Methohexital is a short-acting barbiturate used in ECT that is rapidly metabolized. (Chap. 26)

118. Answer: D

Venlafaxine emerged as a treatment for depression in the 1990s. (Chap. 21)

119. Answer: C

The Columbia Impairment Scale focuses on impairment of function rather than global pathology. (Chap. 28)

120. Answer: C

The study (Lavigne et al., 1998) found that 50% of children who met criteria for a psychiatric disorder in preschool continued to have the disorder 2 years later. (Chap. 45)

121. Answer: D

Erythromycin, sertraline, cimetidine, and aspirin increase valproate levels. (Chap. 22)

122–124. Answers
122-C, 123-B, 124-A.

The Child PTSD Reaction index was the original instrument. The CPTSD-RI and UCLA PTSD Index for DSM-IV are revisions of this. (Chap. 39)

125. Answer: A

Lower doses are associated with more sedation than higher doses of mirtazapine. (Chap. 21)

126. Answer: D

Sertraline alone, CBT alone, CBT plus sertraline, and placebo were compared. Combination treatment, CBT, and sertraline improved outcomes, in that order, with the highest effect size for combination treatment. (Chap. 35)

127. Answer: C

Chronic lithium treatment has been reported in a small number of case reports to cause hyperparathyroidism; therefore, considering checking serum calcium levels annually is a possibility. Renal and thyroid function should be checked every 6 months or when clinically indicated. An ECG is part of the baseline workup and once a therapeutic level has been reached. (Chap. 22)

128. Answer: B

Topiramate has not been shown to be an effective mood stabilizer. (Chap. 22)

129. Answer: C

The fatty acids alpha-linolenic, eicosapentaenoic (EPA), and docosahexaenoic (DHA) are known as omega-3; linoleic and arachidonic acids are known as omega-6. (Chap. 25)

130. Answer: E

The Pediatric Rule of 1998 allowed the FDA to require pediatric studies for certain new and marketed drugs and biological products. Despite the success of the Pediatric Rule, legal challenges arose in 2000 questioning the authority of the FDA (as an agency) to require pharmaceutical companies to conduct pediatric studies under the Pediatric Rule, and a judge ruled the Pediatric Rule invalid. Later legislation by Congress overcame this hurdle. (Chap. 51)

131. Answer: B

Cognitive behavioral therapy with hierarchy-based exposure and response prevention (ERP) has been shown to be a durable treatment for OCD. (Chap. 35)

132. Answer: D

Diagnosis informs the prognosis and the course of illness and delineates empirically validated treatments for that particular disorder. The other elements of an assessment are important for this as well, of course, and also help formulate a diagnosis. (Chap. 27)

133. Answer: D

Depending on the clinical scenario, all of the options are reasonable in treating comorbid ADHD and a tic disorder. (Chap. 36)

134. Answer: C

Ravi Kant et al. in a 2004 report found that clozapine may help control symptoms of bipolar, IED, and PTSD with reduced polypharmacy of mood stabilizers and antidepressants. The use of clozapine is labor-intensive for the patient and family and should be considered carefully. (Chap. 39)

135. Answer: D

$GABA_A$ and $GABA_C$ mediate fast synaptic inhibition via transmitter-gated chloride ion channels. (Chap. 24)

136. Answer: A

A careful exploration for history of bipolar disorder in a family is warranted in the evaluation of a child. (Chap. 33)

137. Answer: A

Tryptophan, an herbal sleep aid, has been associated with eosinophilic myalgia syndrome. (Chap. 46)

138. Answer: C

Benign rashes typically develop within the first 8 weeks of lamotrigine treatment. (Chap. 22)

139. Answer: D

Akathisia has been reported with the use of all second-generation antipsychotics. (Chap. 37)

140. Answer: C

The use of nefazadone led to liver problems in rare instances. (Chap. 21)

141. Answer: B

Schizophrenia and ADHD have been two disorders where dopamine-related alleles have been examined. The findings have not been robust for specific allele effects and studies have had small subject sizes. (Chap. 6)

142. Answer: A

The etiology and physiological reason might be important to know in a given case, but these are not overarching aspects related to decision-making. To the extent possible, the decision-maker must not be proceeding with false expectations; decisions should be congruent with the patient and family's premorbid values and goals. The individual must be able to use reason in the formulation of a choice and communicate that choice to the physician or health-care team. (Chap. 52)

143. Answer: A

There have been deaths from overdoses of SSRIs alone, albeit rare. The evidence does not suggest SSRIs increase suicide completion. (Chap. 20)

144. Answer: B

Serotonin or 5-hydroxytryptamine (5-HT) is produced from tryptophan through hydroxylation and decarboxylation. (Chap. 2)

145. Answer: B

In older surveys dating to 1985, psychiatrists prescribed more than any other group, but this has shifted to pediatricians. (Chap. 49)

146. Answer: B

Oral contraceptives can reduce lamotrigine levels, and abruptly discontinuing the oral contraceptive may lead to a sudden increase in lamotrigine levels, ostensibly increasing the risk for Stevens-Johnson syndrome. (Chap. 27)

147. Answer: C

The specificity is 90%, so the false-positive rate is the remaining percentage. (Chap. 28)

148. Answer: C

Alcohol enhances $GABA_A$ receptor functioning. Benzodiazepines also enhance $GABA_A$ receptor activity, hence their use in alcohol detoxification. (Chap. 2)

149. Answer: B

If the prolactin level is less than 200 ng/mL, the physician can try reducing the dose or switching to a prolactin-sparing drug such as aripiprazole or quetiapine or, in treatment-resistant patients, clozapine. If the level persists with these efforts or if the level is >200 ng/mL, the physician should obtain an MRI of the sella turcica to look for a pituitary adenoma or parasellar tumor. (Chap. 23)

150. Answer: C

Coexisting disorders are present in 50% of patients with childhood-onset schizophrenia. This common occurrence of psychiatric comorbidity probably indicates the severity of underlying neurodevelopmental abnormalities. (Chap. 13)

151. Answer: D

SSRIs down-regulate serotonin receptors, thereby modulating function. Some SSRIs have limited anticholinergic effects rather than cholinergic ones. (Chap. 20)

152. Answer: D

The nonselective, serotonergic and adrenergic, tricyclic clomipramine has been shown to be superior to the SSRIs in pediatric OCD. Its use as a first-line agent is less attractive because of potential side effects and the need for EKGs and blood levels, but it should be considered in more refractory cases. Individual SSRIs appear to have equal efficacy to one another. (Chap. 35)

153. Answer: A

The stimulants are structurally dissimilar but share a phenylethylamine backbone with catecholamines, such as norepinephrine and dopamine. (Chap. 31)

154. Answer: B

There was no placebo arm in the MTA. Community care as usual was the control arm. Behavioral intervention did increase parent/caregiver satisfaction and demonstrated improvement in internalizing symptoms, teacher-rated social skills, reading achievement, and management of comorbid symptoms; for core symptoms of ADHD, stimulants were superior to behavioral intervention and behavioral intervention had no added benefit. (Chap. 18)

155. Answer: E

There is a great variety among individuals in both the number of CYPs and their efficiency. (Chap. 4)

156. Answer: D

The diagnosis of bipolar increased from 25 per 100,000 to 1000 per 100,000, a 40-fold increase. Among those with a new diagnosis (initial diagnosis) of bipolar disorder, most had only one insurance claim for bipolar disorder in the following year after index diagnosis, and only 14% started a mood stabilizer. These findings suggest the diagnosis is often reconsidered or not followed up on by families. (Chap. 49)

157. Answer: D

An effect size of 0.8 is considered large. (Chap. 29)

158. Answer: A

Organogenesis occurs in the first 12 weeks. Medications are considered teratogenic when exposure to the drug during organogenesis results in an increased incidence of birth defects compared with the baseline risk in the general population. (Chap. 44)

159. Answer: A

Phase IV (post-marketing) studies follow up on certain questions or concerns. These might include requests by the FDA for additional efficacy data (e.g., a maintenance study), or if there is a signal for an important safety finding, the FDA might require an additional safety study to explore such a finding. (Chap. 51)

160. Answer: D

Bupropion shares a structure with endogenous amphetamine-like substance, has dopamine and norepinephrine effects, and has been studied in controlled trials to show its effectiveness. (Chap. 31)

161. Answer: B

Medication compliance is not increased. (Chap. 33)

162. Answer: C

10 of 16 subjects assigned to placebo (62.5%) showed significant worsening of irritability symptoms compared with 2 of 16 subjects (12.5%) who continued on risperidone beyond 6 months. (Chap. 38)

163. Answer: B

An EKG can also be considered for patients with cardiac risk factors who are on venlafaxine. (Chap. 21)

164. Answer: E

Posttraumatic stress disorder has not been evaluated in randomized controlled trials of antipsychotics. (Chap. 23)

165. Answer: D

Neural circuit loops in habit formation and tics connect the basal ganglia with the cortex and thalamus. (Chap. 12)

166. Answer: D

An effect size of 0.8 indicates a large effect size for the effectiveness of ECT treatment for certain psychiatric illnesses. (Chap. 26)

167. Answer: C

PATS is the acronym for the Preschool ADHD Treatment Study. (Chap. 45)

168. Answer: A

Thioridazine is avoided because of QTc prolongation. (Chap. 37)

169. Answer: C

Abrupt withdrawal of an antidepressant with REM-suppressing qualities will lead to REM rebound. (Chap. 46)

170. Answer: D

If the public is unaware of the prevalence of childhood psychiatric disorders, the belief that medications are overprescribed might ensue. (Chap. 49)

171. Answer: D

Zolpidem, zaleplon, and eszoplicone all have CYP3A4 metabolism in common. Each agent has additional mechanisms involved its metabolism. (Chap. 24)

172. Answer: B

Growing evidence indicates that untreated symptoms in pregnancy may lead to adverse medical outcomes. (Chap. 44)

173. Answer: C

Gabapentin is reported to cause behavioral disinhibition sometimes in younger children. (Chap. 22)

174. Answer: B

Cognitive behavioral therapy, alone and with motivational enhancement therapy, was also compared. Interpersonal

therapy was not compared. The treatment arms were equally effective. (Chap. 41)

175. Answer: B

The risk is 5% for sisters and 10% for brothers. The risk is 50% for monozygotic twins. (Chap. 12)

176. Answer: D

When switching from an MAOI to another antidepressant, a 2-week drug-free interval is strongly recommended. When switching from one MAOI to another (such as phenelzine), a 2-week drug-free interval is <u>also</u> recommended. (Chap. 21)

177. Answer: B

Antihistamines that are used to help with agitation have anticholinergic properties, and this can be a problem in delirium, cardiac conduction abnormalities, or reactive airway disease. (Chap. 41)

178. Answer: C

Early-morning awakening and "non-restorative" sleep are uncommon complaints in childhood. (Chap. 46)

179. Answer: B

The reaction is the result of increased serotonin and occurs at the receptor site, a physiological effect on the body and hence a pharmacodynamic reaction. (Chap. 4)

180. Answer: C

Manufacturers are responsible for ensuring that a dietary supplement is safe before marketing it. Dietary supplements are not regulated by the FDA but by the Dietary Supplement Health and Education Act (DSHEA). The Federal Trade Commission regulates dietary supplement advertising for false and misleading claims. (Chap. 25)

181. Answer: B

The risk of suicide associated with schizophrenia is highest during the first 10 years of the illness. (Chap. 37)

182. Answer: B

Valproate reaches peak levels after 2 to 4 hours and has a serum half-life between 8 and 16 hours in children and young adolescents. (Chap. 22)

183. Answer: B

Albumin has a high capacity to bind drugs. (Chap. 3)

184. Answer: C

Clonidine is dosed at 3 to 5 micrograms per kilogram per day, with a range of 0.1 to 0.3 milligrams or 100 to 300 micrograms; higher doses have been used when indicated. (Chap. 19)

185. Answer: A

Patients with anorexia have significant bone mineral loss through a number of mechanisms, and at least 1500 mg/day calcium and 400 IU vitamin D should be provided routinely to prevent osteoporosis. (Chap. 40)

186. Answer: A

Splitting the dose does not affect the total dose delivered but reduces the peak concentration. Administering with fatty foods (rather than without) will also reduce peak levels. (Chap. 23)

187. Answer: D

For patients stabilized on lithium the risk of relapse was high with noncompliance, although noncompliance can be a marker for other factors contributing to illness. (Chap. 33)

188. Answer: C

A fourth of the industry's revenue, which equaled $57.5 billion, was spent on promotion and advertising, three-fourths of which was spent on advertising campaigns in journals, professional meetings, and direct contact with physicians. (Chap. 30)

189. Answer: B

The licensing requirements of the Drug Enforcement Agency would not be an area that is germane. (Chap. 49)

190. Answer: D

Modern ECT uses "brief pulse" machines that typically use a pulse width of 0.5 to 2 milliseconds, although emerging research may indicate the effectiveness of even briefer pulse widths. (Chap. 26)

191. Answer: C

Data Monitoring Committees (DMC), also known as Data Monitoring Review Boards (DSMB), monitor ongoing clinical drug trials. (Chap. 52)

192. Answer: D

Only fluoxetine, however, is FDA-approved for childhood depression. (Chap. 32)

193. Answer: A

A resting pulse of 60 bpm, blood pressure measures that are two standard deviations from gender and age means on two repeat evaluations, and orthostatic blood pressure and pulse changes of 10% or greater should lead to further exploration. (Chap. 19)

194. Answer: C

Brain areas involved in the stress response also modulate motor behavior, affect regulation, arousal, sleep, startle response, attention, and cardiovascular function, so it is not unusual for children to present with symptoms of ADHD. Option B is a statement without giving a reason. Option D has some potential validity but is a generalization about children with PTSD. (Chap. 39)

195. Answer: B

Clonidine was first used in the treatment of hypertension and was subsequently used in tic disorders and ADHD. (Chap. 19)

196. Answer: B

A screening instrument rated by a panel of experts for its relevance to a construct being measured refers to content validity. (Chap. 28)

197. Answer: D

The capability of recognizing biological motion emerges very early in development, indicating that this capacity is significant for social engagement. (Chap. 14)

198. Answer: C

Compulsions and obsessions need not accompany one another. (Chap. 35)

199. Answer: E

Language skills and adaptive skills are strong predictors of eventual outcome. (Chap. 38)

200. Answer: B

Methylphenidate and clonidine were both effective for ADHD, with stimulants having a larger effect size. (Chap. 18)

Test 3 Questions

1. With a dopamine antagonist, what dopamine receptor occupancy is needed for antipsychotic efficacy?

    A. 10% to 25%

    B. 25% to 40%

    C. 40% to 60%

    D. 60% to 75%

2. Which of the following effects of trazodone results in the potential for priapism as an adverse effect?

    A. Serotonin agonism

    B. Antihistaminergic effects

    C. Peripheral alpha-adrenergic antagonism

    D. Anticholinergic effects

3. All of the following foods can promote pediatric constipation EXCEPT:

    A. Milk products

    B. Chocolate

    C. Caffeinated beverages

    D. High-fructose corn syrup

4. What is the male-to-female sex ratio for the incidence of Rett's disorder?

    A. 2 to 1

    B. 1 to 3

    C. 1 to 4

    D. 1 to 6

    E. None of the above

5. Maternal panic disorder during pregnancy has been associated with an increased risk for developing:

    A. Preterm labor

    B. Pre-eclampsia

    C. Placental abruption

    D. Gestational diabetes

6. Which of the following most resembles paternalism?

    A. Autonomy

    B. Justice

    C. Nonmaleficence

    D. Beneficence

7. Youths suffering from major depressive disorder (MDD) with psychotic symptoms have an increased risk for all the following outcomes EXCEPT:

    A. More severe depression

    B. Greater long-term morbidity

    C. Bipolar disorder

    D. Dysthymic disorder

8. What is the first step in the treatment of posttraumatic stress disorder (PTSD)?

    A. Psychoeducation

    B. Trauma-focused CBT (TF-CBT)

    C. Cognitive behavioral therapy

    D. Exposure and response prevention

9. In a group of adolescent patients with substance use disorder and various bipolar diagnoses, which of the following was found to statistically reduce the number of positive urine screens?

    A. Olanzapine

    B. Valproic acid

    C. Lithium

    D. Fluoxetine

10. Which of the following agents has been shown to be effective in clinical trials for attention-deficit/hyperactivity disorder but was not approved for ADHD because of the presence of a number of Stevens-Johnson–like rashes in trials?

    A. Bupropion

    B. Clonidine

    C. Nortriptyline

    D. Modafinil

11. A 14-year-old boy on 200 milligrams of lamotrigine daily has recently started receiving adjunct valproate treatment due to severe symptoms of mania. What other intervention might be considered?

    A. Increasing the dose of lamotrigine

    B. Maintaining the dose of lamotrigine

    C. Decreasing the dose of lamotrigine

    D. Discontinuing lamotrigine treatment

12. Which of the following is a side effect of pregabalin?

    A. Weight loss

    B. Sialorrhea

    C. Somnolence

    D. Hyperfocus

13. SLITRK1 candidate gene is thought to contribute to the development of which of the following in Tourette's disorder?

    A. Dopamine receptor sensitivity

    B. Dopamine neuronal re-uptake

    C. Cortico-striatal-thalamic-cortical circuits

    D. Radial glial cell migration

14. In adults, which cognitive deficit arising from electroconvulsive therapy (ECT) is of the most concern?

    A. Dyscalculia

    B. Retrograde amnesia

    C. Dysphasia

    D. Anterograde amnesia

15. Approximately how much time does it take to establish the steady state of a drug?

    A. 2 times the half-life

    B. 3 times the half-life

    C. 4 times the half-life

    D. 5 times the half-life

    E. 10 times the half-life

16. True or False. Due to lithium's action on antidiuretic hormone in the distal tubules and collecting ducts, the development of diabetes insipidus can be irreversible.

    A. True

    B. False

17. The TWO most important factors affecting the volume of distribution of a drug in the body are:

    A. Fat stores

    B. Rate of absorption

    C. Relative proportion of total body water to extracellular water

    D. Intracellular water

18. Treatment of which of the following has been shown to prevent the onset of depressive disorders in children?

    A. Falling academic performance

    B. Decreasing social participation

    C. Parental depression

    D. Posttraumatic stress symptoms

19. According to National Ambulatory Medical Care Survey data, the rate of antipsychotic prescribing in children and adolescents from 1993 to 2002:

    A. Decreased

    B. Remained the same

    C. Increased 2-fold

    D. Increased 6-fold

20. What is the rate of comorbid psychiatric disorders in adolescents with substance use disorders?

    A. 5%

    B. 25%

    C. 35%

    D. 75%

21. Which of the following is true about seizure activity and aggressive behavior?

    A. Aggression during the interictal period is usually non-directed and unintentional.

    B. A correlation between criminal activity and seizure activity has been demonstrated.

    C. Incarcerated individuals have a two- to four-fold higher rate of epilepsy.

    D. Aggression during the ictal period is in response to a social context.

22. Children who have bipolar disorder and co-occurring anxiety disorders compared with those who have bipolar disorder alone manifest all the following EXCEPT:

    A. Manic symptoms at an earlier age

    B. Higher likelihood of hospitalization

    C. Increased treatment non-adherence

    D. Poorer outcome

For the following four questions, match who is typically the best informant for specific symptoms suffered during a developmental stage.

23. Rating a child's capacity for sustained attention

24. Rating a young child's sleep disturbance

25. Rating a school-age child's anxiety

26. Rating symptoms of conduct disorder or substance use

    A. The child patient

    B. Teacher

    C. Parent

    D. The adolescent patient

27. Which of the following is the type of question that pragmatic clinical trials seek to answer?

    A. Does this intervention work under usual conditions?

    B. Does this intervention work under ideal conditions?

    C. Both statements

    D. None of the above

28. Which of the following physicochemical properties of a drug would likely result in reduced absorption?

    A. Non-polar, highly lipid-soluble, and small molecular size

    B. Non-polar, non-lipid-soluble, and medium molecular size

    C. Highly polar, non-lipid-soluble, and large molecular size

    D. None of the above

29. What percentage of children experience resolution of nocturnal enuresis when prescribed desmopressin acetate?

    A. 10%

    B. 20%

    C. 50%

    D. 70%

30. What is the female-to-male ratio of depression occurrence in younger children?

    A. 1 to 1

    B. 2 to 1

    C. 3 to 1

    D. 4 to 1

31. Dopaminergic neurons from the hypothalamus project primarily to which brain area?

    A. Caudate and putamen

    B. Nucleus accumbens and amygdala

    C. Frontal, cingulate, and entorhinal cortex

    D. Pituitary gland

32. In the clinically meaningful metric of effect size, a small magnitude of effect is represented by which of the following decimals?

    A. 0.3

    B. 0.5

    C. 0.7

    D. 0.9

33. Which area of the brain has a highly selective role in processing faces over any other category of visual stimuli?

    A. Dorsolateral prefrontal cortex

    B. Lateral fusiform gyrus

    C. Entorhinal cortex

    D. Subthalamic nucleus

34. If a patient complains of gastrointestinal symptoms, gains 7% or more of their baseline body weight, or has an increase of 0.5 in the BMI z-score when treated for >3 months on an antipsychotic, which labs might be obtained?

    A. Prolactin

    B. CBC

    C. AST, ALT, or GGT

    D. Electrolytes

35. Which TWO brain structures compose the medial temporal lobe?

    A. Hippocampus

    B. Hypothalamus

    C. Amygdala

    D. Thalamus

36. Which is the most accurate statement about stimulants in childhood posttraumatic stress disorder (PTSD)?

    A. They should not be used because they can lead to affective dysregulation.

    B. They should not be used because they worsen hyperarousal symptoms.

    C. They may help symptoms of hyperactivity and inattention attributable to PTSD.

    D. They may help symptoms of avoidance and numbing by enhancing motivation.

37. Which type of monoamine oxidase predominates in the CNS?

    A. Monoamine oxidase-A (MAO-A)

    B. Monoamine oxidase-B (MAO-B)

    C. Both are equally prevalent.

    D. None of the above

38. Which of the following should be explored and is most prevalent in overweight youths?

    A. Somatization disorders

    B. Binge eating disorder

    C. Separation anxiety disorder

    D. Prader-Willi syndrome

39. The likelihood of mixed-episode bipolar disorder in children compared with adults is:

    A. Equivalent

    B. Increased

    C. Decreased

    D. Not present in children

40. Which of the following agents has been studied in the treatment of Alzheimer's disease and dementia, so far with negative results?

    A. Gingko biloba

    B. S-adenosyl methionine

    C. St. John's wort

    D. Kava

    E. Secretin

41. When a drug eliminated by first-order kinetics is dosed at regular intervals what parameter determines the plasma steady-state concentration?

    A. Clearance

    B. Plasma half-life

    C. Absorption

    D. Bioavailability

42. In acute anorexia nervosa, weight loss causes:

    A. Hypoleptinemia

    B. Hyperleptinemia

    C. No change in leptin levels

    D. Leptin is not related to body weight change.

43. Research into pharmacogenomic testing to determine polymorphisms that may help guide selective serotonin reuptake inhibitor (SSRI) dosing and administration has focused on all of the following EXCEPT:

    A. Cytochrome P450 isoenzymes

    B. The promoter region of the serotonin transporter

    C. Postsynaptic serotonin receptors

    D. Enzymes of the serotonin synthetic pathway

    E. Serotonin vesicle release

44. Buspirone has been shown to reduce which of the following?

    A. SSRI-induced sexual dysfunction

    B. SSRI-induced suicidal thinking

    C. SSRI-induced bleeding

    D. SSRI-induced tremors

45. What is citalopram's half-life in adolescents?

    A. 5 hours

    B. 10 hours

    C. 40 hours

    D. 5 days

    E. 10 days

46. All the following statements are accurate EXCEPT:

    A. Carbamazepine's P450 drug interactions make its clinical use difficult.

    B. Carbamazepine's autoinduction requires increased dosing to maintain initial levels.

    C. There is good evidence for the use of carbamazepine as a first-line agent for children and adolescents with bipolar disorder.

    D. Carbamazepine can be considered in bipolar disorder if a child fails to respond to other treatment regimens.

47. Which of the following would be an acceptable approach to treating severe pediatric anxiety?

    A. Cognitive behavioral therapy alone

    B. SSRI alone

    C. Combination SSRI and cognitive behavioral therapy

    D. All of the above

48. Which of the following is the primary reason to consider prescribing medication for tics?

    A. The tics interfere with the child's life.

    B. Anti-tic medication improves the course and severity of the illness.

    C. The parents request it.

    D. All of the above

49. Which of the following is *generally* the preferred order of treatment in an individual with the following co-occurring illnesses?

    A. Treat mania>ADHD>depression.

    B. Treat ADHD>mania>depression.

    C. Treat depression>mania>ADHD.

    D. Treat depression>ADHD>mania.

For the following questions, match the drug with the correct FDA labeling for children and/or adolescents. A drug may have more than one correct corresponding answer option, or an answer option may correspond to more than one drug.

50. Lithium

51. Trifluoperazine

52. Quetiapine

53. Olanzapine

    A. Approved for the treatment of schizophrenia

    B. Approved for "psychotic children," aged 6 to 12

    C. Approved for the treatment of bipolar I disorder (may be for manic or mixed/manic)

    D. Labeling indicates that safety and effectiveness in patients with mania below the age of 12 years have not been established, thereby implying that data are available down to age 12 years.

54. What does "pharmacogenomics" refer to?

    A. An area of research that employs genetic information in drug design and treatment

    B. An area of research that uses stem cell DNA to design drugs

    C. An area of research that uses drug actions to determine genetic function

    D. An area of research that uses the body's own proteins for drug development

55. Pregabalin has FDA indications for which conditions?

    A. Management of neuropathic pain

    B. Post-herpetic neuralgia

    C. Partial-onset seizures

    D. All of the above

56. Which of the following is the slow-acting postsynaptic receptor?

    A. Ionotropic receptor

    B. G-protein-coupled receptor

    C. Autoreceptor

    D. Heteroreceptor

57. All of these are anticholinergic effects of antihistamines EXCEPT:

    A. Dry mouth

    B. Cough

    C. Dysuria

    D. Incontinence

    E. Delirium

58. Carbamazepine is slowly absorbed from the gastrointestinal system and is:

    A. Highly bioavailable

    B. Poorly bioavailable

    C. Highly protein bound

    D. Poorly protein bound

    E. A and C

59. In which of the following illnesses has vagus nerve stimulation (VNS) been proven effective?

    A. Bipolar disorder

    B. Intractable anxiety disorders

    C. Treatment-resistant depression

    D. Refractory epilepsy

60. What was a significant change in pediatric psychopharmacology towards the turn of the 21st century?

    A. The emergence of risperidone and other atypical antipsychotics

    B. The emergence of methylphenidate

    C. The emergence of federally sponsored, large multi-site studies

    D. The recognition that children suffer from mental illness

61. Approximately what percentage of patients with childhood-onset schizophrenia have smooth pursuit eye movement abnormalities?

    A. 15%

    B. 25%

    C. 60%

    D. 80%

62. In a clinical trial, in addition to the group mean change in the continuous measurement of the primary outcome variable, it is informative to report:

    A. The dollar amount spent on the trial

    B. The primary investigator's history of clinical trial experience

    C. The patients' perspectives on the trial experience

    D. The rate of responders in each treatment group

63. The neurocognitive sequelae of childhood cancers may benefit from which treatment?

    A. Fluoxetine

    B. Citalopram

    C. Methylphenidate

    D. Clonidine

64. What does the evidence suggest regarding the use of risperidone in pediatric patients with comorbid epilepsy?

    A. Risperidone reduces the frequency of seizures.

    B. Risperidone increases the frequency of seizures.

    C. Risperidone has no effect on seizures.

    D. Risperidone is contraindicated.

65. Which of the following statements about valproate is TRUE?

    A. It is highly protein-bound.

    B. It binds poorly to proteins.

    C. It is metabolized in the liver.

    D. It is metabolized by the kidneys.

    E. A and C

66. Which is true about CYP polymorphisms?

    A. There are no gender differences.

    B. There are gender differences.

    C. CYP1A2 is more active in females.

    D. CYP2D6 is more active in males.

67. What is the age of onset for selective mutism?

    A. 0 to 24 months

    B. 2 to 5 years

    C. 5 to 8 years

    D. >8 years

68. Approximately what percentage of substance use disorders begin in childhood or adolescence?

    A. 1% to 2%

    B. 10% to 17%

    C. 30% to 50%

    D. >50%

69. Which term describes the possibility that a parent may rate his or her child on a screening instrument in overly positive or negative terms?

    A. Face validity

    B. Content validity

    C. Positive predictive power

    D. "Halo" effect

70. After a drug company has completed its drug development program through clinical trials and the drug has shown positive results, what may happen next?

    A. Submission of data to the Centers for Disease Control

    B. Submission of New Drug Application

    C. Submission of Investigational New Drug Application

    D. Submission of marketing materials to the FDA

71. A meta-analysis of studies of mostly adult patients looking at pharmacologic treatment for generalized anxiety disorder (GAD) found what effect size for selective serotonin reuptake inhibitors (SSRIs)?

    A. 0.36

    B. 0.86

    C. 1.66

    D. There was no effect.

72. Although the distinction between atypical and typical antipsychotics can be arbitrary, what is the advantage of using an atypical antipsychotic?

    A. Less weight gain

    B. Less sedation

    C. Less risk of tardive dyskinesia

    D. More effective

73. A meta-analysis found that ECT had what magnitude of effect size on the basis of six randomized sham-ECT controlled trials involving 256 patients?

    A. 0.91

    B. 0.62

    C. 0.38

    D. 0.16

74. All the following are common adverse effects of clonidine EXCEPT:

    A. Dry mouth

    B. Dizziness

    C. Fatigue

    D. Weakness

    E. Asymptomatic 10% drop in blood pressure

75. Oxcarbazepine, which is biotransformed by hydroxylation to its active metabolite, is an analogue of:

    A. Imipramine

    B. Olanzapine

    C. Asenapine

    D. Carbamazepine

    E. Topiramate

76. Individual randomized clinical trials as well as a meta-analysis have shown what comparative efficacy of tricyclic antidepressants (TCAs) versus placebo for the treatment of pediatric major depression?

    A. Greater efficacy

    B. Decreased efficacy

    C. Equivalent efficacy

    D. None of the above

77. Which of the following tricyclic antidepressants is FDA-approved for obsessive-compulsive disorder in children older than 10 years?

    A. Imipramine

    B. Clomipramine

    C. Doxepin

    D. Amitriptyline

78. Larger studies with enough statistical power to test specific hypotheses about treatment efficacy in a randomized and conclusive way are called:

    A. Phase 0 trials

    B. Phase I trials

    C. Phase II trials

    D. Phase III trials

    E. Phase IV trials

79. When is the muscle relaxant administered in electroconvulsive therapy (ECT)?

    A. Prior to the administration of the anesthetic agent

    B. Concurrent to the administration of the anesthetic agent

    C. Subsequent to the administration of the anesthetic agent

    D. A muscle relaxant is not administered in ECT.

80. With the exception of the $5HT_3$ receptor, all serotonin receptors are:

    A. Composed of six subunits

    B. Ionic receptors

    C. G-protein-coupled receptors

    D. A and C

81. Muscarinic receptors bind which of the following compounds?

    A. Acetylcholine

    B. Muscarine

    C. Pilocarpine

    D. All of the above

82. The alpha-2 agonists improve prefrontal cortex (PFC) functioning by mimicking which neurotransmitter?

    A. Dopamine

    B. Norepinephrine

    C. Serotonin

    D. Glutamate

83. Which surface of the prefrontal cortex (PFC) uses working memory to guide movement and attention?

    A. Dorsal PFC

    B. Lateral PFC

    C. Ventromedial PFC

    D. A and B

84. Two to five drug-free weeks are strongly recommended when switching from a selective serotonin reuptake inhibitor (SSRI) to which medication?

    A. Nortriptyline

    B. Tranylcypromine

    C. Bupropion

    D. Duloxetine

85. What is the prevalence of elimination disorders in North American school-age children?

    A. 1% to 2%

    B. 2% to 7%

    C. 17% to 29%

    D. 39% to 51%

86. Which of the following is the most common child psychiatric disorder presenting to pediatricians, mental health workers, and child psychiatrists?

    A. Attention-deficit/hyperactivity disorder

    B. Major depressive disorder

    C. Bipolar disorder, not otherwise specified

    D. Schizophrenia

    E. Generalized anxiety disorder

87. **What kind of receptor found in the hippocampus is important for long-term potentiation, a crucial component in the formation of memory?**

    A. NMDA receptor

    B. Alpha-2 receptor

    C. AMPA receptor

    D. GABA receptor

88. **Which is the most prevalent childhood disorder in the community?**

    A. Major depressive disorder

    B. Anxiety disorder

    C. Bipolar disorder

    D. Attention-deficit/hyperactivity disorder

89. **All of the following have at least one randomized controlled trial showing effectiveness for aggression in youth EXCEPT:**

    A. Quetiapine

    B. Divalproex sodium

    C. Olanzapine

    D. Iloperidone

90. **Which of the following symptoms manifesting in a patient on an antipsychotic increases the risk of tardive dyskinesia?**

    A. Parkinsonian symptoms

    B. Akathisia

    C. Dystonic symptoms

    D. A and C

91. **What is a crossover design in a clinical trial?**

    A. Subjects are assigned randomly to one treatment of two or more alternatives.

    B. Subjects are given sequentially and in random order all the treatments that are being tested.

    C. Subjects are assigned randomly to active treatment.

    D. Subjects are assigned to treatment as usual.

92. **Alpha-2 heteroreceptors do which of the following?**

    A. Inhibit the release of dopamine

    B. Enhance the release of dopamine

    C. Inhibit the release of dopamine and glutamate

    D. Enhance the release of dopamine and serotonin

93. **How does hypoleptinemia in anorexia contribute to bone density loss?**

    A. Deactivation of the hypothalamus-pituitary axis

    B. Hypercortisolism

    C. Increase in thyroid-stimulating hormone

    D. Enhancement of renal function

94. **Many of the studies of disorder association and pharmacogenetics of serotonin alleles have examined:**

    A. Fluoxetine

    B. Perfusion effects in the prefrontal cortex

    C. 5-HTPLPR

    D. Tryptophan levels in the central nervous system

95. **Which of the following does the American Academy of Child and Adolescent Psychiatry recommend in mild or moderate cases of obsessive-compulsive disorder?**

    A. Pharmacotherapy

    B. Combination of cognitive behavioral therapy and pharmacotherapy

    C. Cognitive behavioral therapy

    D. Supportive therapy

96. **Amantadine is a noncompetitive antagonist of which of the following receptors?**

    A. GABA

    B. NMDA

    C. NE

    D. DA

    E. 5-HT

97. **In Expert Consensus and Clinicians' Consensus surveys, which atypical antipsychotic was rated most helpful in the treatment of patients with severe and persistent physical aggression and those who destroyed property?**

    A. Olanzapine

    B. Risperidone

    C. Quetiapine

    D. Aripiprazole

98. Fluvoxamine inhibits cytochrome P450 enzymes. Which of the following is the correct order of inhibition from weak to significant?

    A. 1A2, 3A4, 2C9, 2C19, 2D6

    B. 2D6, 1A2, 3A4, 2C9, 2C19

    C. 1A2, 2D6, 3A4, 2C9, 2C19

    D. 2D6, 2C19, 2C9, 3A4, 1A2

99. Parkinsonian symptoms and acute dystonia from antipsychotic treatment occur in youths how frequently compared with adults?

    A. Less frequently

    B. Just as frequently

    C. More frequently

    D. Do not occur

100. Which of the following tools have been developed for parent and teacher ratings of children with intellectual disability?

    A. Aberrant Behavior Checklist (ABC)

    B. Nisonger Child Behavior Rating Form (NCBRF)

    C. Scale of Hostility and Aggression: Reactive/ Proactive (SHARP)

    D. All of the above

101. Which of the following conditions would be an absolute contraindication for electroconvulsive therapy (ECT)?

    A. Recent myocardial infarct

    B. Recent stroke

    C. Unstable coronary syndrome

    D. None of the above

102. What happens in preclinical testing of a new drug?

    A. Healthy volunteer randomized trial

    B. Animal testing

    C. Healthy volunteer dose study

    D. Phase 0 trial

103. What is a side effect of prolactin elevation?

    A. Alopecia

    B. Decreased expression of breast milk

    C. Decreased libido

    D. Increased menstrual bleeding

104. The frequency of serious rashes associated with lamotrigine treatment is approximately what percentage in children less than 16 years old?

    A. 0.01%

    B. 0.25%

    C. 1%

    D. 5%

    E. 10%

105. What is one of the problems with "whistle blowing"?

    A. It costs money.

    B. It helps bring misdeeds to light.

    C. Whistle blowing is unethical.

    D. Reputations can be damaged if whistle blowing is conducted hastily.

106. What is the mechanism of action of atomoxetine?

    A. Specific norepinephrine reuptake inhibitor

    B. Specific serotonin reuptake inhibitor

    C. Specific dopamine reuptake inhibitor

    D. Norepinephrine and dopamine reuptake inhibitor

107. Preschool children with disruptive behavior disorders appear to have approximately what percentage of risk for developing an additional psychiatric disorder within 3 years?

    A. 5%

    B. 20%

    C. 70%

    D. 90%

108. What is a finding of the 8-year prospective follow-up of the Multimodal Treatment Study for ADHD (MTA)?

    A. Long-term data do not demonstrate any advantage to having received initial assignment to the medication arm of the controlled, 14-month phase of the study.

    B. Initial clinical presentation in childhood appears to be the best predictor of later adolescent functioning, rather than the specific treatment received.

    C. After the first 14 months of this study, care was no longer provided by the study team and children returned to care in the community to pursue treatment as desired.

    D. 38.5% of the children receiving medications at 14 months were still taking medication at the 8-year follow-up.

    E. All of the above

109. Which of the following may be a sign of an eating disorder?

    A. Posttraumatic stress disorder

    B. Eating a nutritiously balanced meal

    C. Eating separately from the family

    D. Eating a high-calorie dessert before the main meal

110. During adolescence, for children with early-onset schizophrenia spectrum disorders (EOSS), hallucinations become predominantly auditory. Which types of hallucinations are present in earlier years?

    A. Auditory

    B. Visual

    C. Tactile

    D. All of the above

111. The clinical effect after ingestion of amphetamine and methylphenidate is present as soon as:

    A. 5 to 10 minutes

    B. 30 minutes

    C. 60 minutes

    D. 90 minutes

112. Which of the following monoamine oxidase enzymes preferentially metabolizes serotonin, norepinephrine, and epinephrine?

    A. Monoamine oxidase A (MAO-A)

    B. Monoamine oxidase B (MAO-B)

    C. Both A and B

    D. None of the above

113. The norepinephrine transporter (NET) is the primary route of removal of norepinephrine from the synapse. Which drug(s) selectively block the NET?

    A. Desipramine

    B. Amphetamine

    C. Methylphenidate

    D. B and C

114. What is the incidence of major birth defects in the United States?

    A. 0.5% to 1%

    B. 1% to 2%

    C. 2% to 4%

    D. 5% to 10%

115. Family-Focused Treatment for Adolescents (FFT-A) is a psychosocial intervention based on the finding that bipolar patients who have families with high expressed emotions have which of the following?

    A. Comorbid substance use disorders

    B. Poor treatment response

    C. Increased rate of suicide

    D. High relapse rates

    E. B and C

116. Which of the following is available as a transdermal patch?

    A. Risperidone

    B. Lisdexamfetamine

    C. Clonidine

    D. Guanfacine

117. A brain structure critical to drug-seeking behaviors in addicted-animal studies is the:

    A. Amygdala

    B. Prefrontal cortex

    C. Nucleus accumbens

    D. Locus coeruleus

118. The phenomenon of ultradian cycling in bipolar disorder consists of mood disturbance that meet criteria for a manic, mixed, hypomanic, or major depressive episode in what frequency?

    A. Four or more cycles per year

    B. 5 to 364 cycles per year

    C. Greater than 365 cycles per year

    D. None of the above

119. Which of the following is a specific alpha-2a agonist?

    A. Clonidine

    B. Loratadine

    C. Guanfacine

    D. Mirtazapine

120. A child presents for a given office visit with a diagnosis of attention-deficit/hyperactivity disorder (ADHD). He is more likely to leave the office with a prescription if he or she was seen by a:

    A. Psychiatrist

    B. Pediatrician

    C. Family practitioner

    D. Advanced practice registered nurse (APRN)

121. Which statement best describes respiratory depression and benzodiazepine administration?

    A. Respiratory depression is common at therapeutic doses.

    B. Respiratory depression is more common in healthy young adult males.

    C. Benzodiazepines do not appear to cause depression even at high doses.

    D. Ethanol in moderate doses reduces the risk of respiratory depression.

122. A decrease in which of the following kinds of sleep may lead to subjective feeling of "non-restorative" sleep or not feeling well rested?

    A. Slow-wave sleep

    B. REM sleep

    C. Sleep induction

    D. Parasomnias

123. Bupropion is NOT recommended for patients with which of the following conditions?

    A. Bulimia nervosa

    B. Uncontrolled diabetes mellitus

    C. Major depressive disorder

    D. A and B

124. A review of eight controlled, double-blind studies on the effectiveness of imipramine for enuresis revealed relapse rates following treatment at what percentage?

    A. 35%

    B. 55%

    C. 75%

    D. 90%

125. What agents have had some success in producing weight loss in pediatric patients prescribed antipsychotics?

    A. Metformin, topiramate, amantadine, and orlistat

    B. Stimulants and topiramate

    C. Fluoxetine

    D. No agents have proved useful.

126. The Food and Drug Administration mandated a black box warning for stimulants for which of the following?

    A. Manic symptoms

    B. Insomnia

    C. Gastrointestinal distress

    D. Abuse potential

127. Which one of the following instruments, which have all been used to determine symptom outcomes in clinical trials for children or adolescents with depression, is clinician-administered?

    A. Beck Depression Inventory (BDI

    B. Children's Depression Rating Scale, Revised (CDRS-Revised)

    C. Children's Depression Inventory (CDI)

    D. Center for Epidemiological Studies Depression Scale (CES-D)

    E. All of the above

128. How long should a medication for a first episode of pediatric obsessive-compulsive disorder (OCD) be continued?

    A. 6 to 12 months after stabilization

    B. 6 to 12 months after initiation

    C. 1 to 2 years after stabilization

    D. Until adolescence

129. Currently all stimulants used to treat attention-deficit/hyperactivity disorder (ADHD) and atomoxetine carry detailed warning language to alert prescribers and consumers of a potential association with:

    A. Sudden cardiac death in the context of a shift in heart rate or blood pressure

    B. Liver failure when stimulants and atomoxetine are taken concurrently

    C. Pulmonary hypertension in the context of excessive exercise

    D. Sudden cardiac death in the presence of underlying structural heart disease or family history of such disease

130. Growing empirical data link a strong alliance in pharmacotherapy with which kind of clinical outcome?

    A. Negative

    B. Positive

    C. No association with either negative or positive outcome

    D. Positive effect up to a point, then detrimental

131. Duloxetine is FDA-approved for which of the following indications?

    A. Social phobia

    B. Diabetic peripheral neuropathy

    C. Fibromyalgia

    D. B and C

132. Which of the following medications is approved for use as a hypnotic in children by the Food and Drug Administration?

    A. Zaleplon

    B. Trazodone

    C. Lorazepam

    D. None

133. The surface area of the human cortex is how many times larger than that of the monkey?

    A. 100-fold

    B. 50-fold

    C. 20-fold

    D. 10-fold

    E. 5-fold

134. All the following factors in a child's history and presentation raise suspicion for possible bipolar disorder EXCEPT:

    A. Episodic mood lability

    B. Developmental delay

    C. Antidepressant-induced mania

    D. Early-onset depression

135. Which of the following agents would be avoided as a first-line treatment for attention-deficit/ hyperactivity disorder (ADHD) in substance-abusing youths?

    A. Stimulants

    B. Guanfacine

    C. Atomoxetine

    D. Bupropion

136. Olanzapine has been shown to increase which of the following physiological indicators?

    A. Fasting glucose

    B. Fasting total cholesterol

    C. Fasting triglycerides

    D. All of the above

137. Separation anxiety disorder typically develops during which stage?

    A. Preschool years

    B. Latency years

    C. Adolescence

    D. Adulthood

138. What is the usual number of sessions for electro-convulsive therapy (ECT) in adults?

    A. 2 to 6

    B. 6 to 12

    C. 12 to 18

    D. 18 to 24

139. Omega-3 supplementation for depression in children has been examined. Which option accurately represents the present number of randomized controlled trials conducted in children?

    A. 1

    B. 6

    C. 12

    D. 18

140. Why do open-label trials almost always show greater benefit than the subsequent large randomized trials?

    A. There is no correction for placebo.

    B. Raters are not blinded.

    C. Subjects are aware of the treatment.

    D. The clinical scale thresholds for pathology are set differently.

141. The diagnostic criterion in anorexia nervosa of body weight maintenance below 85% of expected weight corresponds to what percentile of body mass index (BMI)?

    A. 2%

    B. 5%

    C. 10%

    D. 20%

142. A recent study of a population-based birth cohort of preschool-age children (N = 1950) whose developmental trajectories of hyperactivity were assessed between the ages of 17 and 41 months found that frequent hyperactivity was related specifically to deficits in which neurocognitive trait?

    A. Expressive language

    B. Receptive language

    C. Visuospatial organization

    D. Fine motor skills

143. What is the appropriate dose of diphenhydramine in a pediatric patient who is agitated?

    A. 25 to 50 mg

    B. 100 to 150 mg

    C. 200 mg

    D. Diphenhydramine should not be used because it can lead to paradoxical disinhibition.

144. A large double-blind, placebo-controlled, parallel assignment trial to study the effect of fluoxetine for reducing repetitive behaviors in autism resulted in what preliminary outcome?

    A. Fluoxetine was significantly better than placebo in reducing repetitive behaviors.

    B. Fluoxetine was no better than placebo in reducing repetitive behaviors.

    C. A dose–response relationship determines the effect of fluoxetine on repetitive behaviors.

    D. The placebo was significantly better than fluoxetine in reducing repetitive behaviors.

145. Over 80 obsessive-compulsive disorder (OCD) candidate gene studies have been reported over the past decade. The candidate genes have been selected for their putative role in neurotransmitter pathways or anatomy believed to be involved in OCD. Which neurotransmitter system gene is the only one to have been consistently replicated?

    A. Serotonin

    B. Glutamate

    C. Dopamine

    D. Histamine

    E. Acetylcholine

146. What percentage of all drugs is metabolized by CYP-450?

    A. Up to 30%

    B. Up to 50%

    C. Up to 70%

    D. Up to 90%

147. In the treatment of anorexia nervosa, which of the following statements is most accurate based on the evidence?

    A. Family work is more successful if held in conjoint sessions of adolescent and parent together when there is a high degree of conflict.

    B. Family work is more successful if held in separate adolescent and parent sessions when there is a high degree of conflict.

    C. Non-intact families benefit from a shorter duration of treatment.

    D. When comorbid disorders are present, the treatment of anorexia should be deferred.

148. What does the data suggest about increased suicidal thinking on selective serotonin reuptake inhibitors (SSRIs) in pooled pediatric obsessive-compulsive disorder (OCD) trials?

    A. There is a statistically significant increase in suicidal thinking on SSRIs.

    B. There is no statistically significant increase in suicidal thinking on SSRIs.

    C. There are three reported suicides during pediatric OCD trials.

    D. There is a decrease in suicidal thinking on SSRIs.

149. Mirtazapine has synergistic depressant effects on motor and cognitive performance when used in conjunction with:

    A. Benzodiazepines

    B. Selective serotonin reuptake inhibitors (SSRIs)

    C. Alcohol

    D. A and C

150. Which drug might be useful for chronic pain of unknown etiology and major depressive disorder?

    A. Gabapentin

    B. Naltrexone

    C. Duloxetine

    D. Naproxen

151. Alpha-2 receptor stimulation in the prefrontal cortex results in:

    A. Enhanced functioning

    B. Reduced functioning

    C. No change

    D. There are no alpha-2 receptors in the prefrontal cortex.

152. Which of the following statements is most accurate?

    A. Obtaining an ECG is advised before starting children on clonidine.

    B. Obtaining an ECG, blood pressure, and pulse is advised before starting children on clonidine.

    C. Obtaining a blood pressure and pulse is advised before starting children on clonidine.

    D. A blood pressure, pulse, or ECG is not usually obtained before starting children on clonidine.

153. What are the most common obsessions in children ages 6 to 17?

    A. Sexual obsessions

    B. Religious obsessions

    C. Food obsessions

    D. Harm obsessions

154. There have been four randomized controlled trials of lithium for pediatric aggression. Which statement captures the state of the evidence?

    A. There have been one positive trial and three negative trials.

    B. There have been two positive trials and two negative trials.

    C. All trials were positive.

    D. All trials were negative.

155. Collectively, the selective serotonin reuptake inhibitors do not have strong evidence for use in childhood posttraumatic stress disorder (PTSD), although they have the potential to ameliorate all symptom clusters in PTSD. They may be more effective than other agents for which symptom cluster in particular?

    A. Re-experiencing

    B. Avoidance and numbing

    C. Hyperarousal

    D. Somatic

156. Lesions in which brain area generally increase aggression?

    A. Parietal cortex

    B. Prefrontal cortex

    C. Cerebellum

    D. Occipital cortex

157. Retrospective studies of adults with bipolar disorder have found what percentage reporting that their illness started before age 19?

    A. 5% to 18%

    B. 15% to 26%

    C. 23% to 50%

    D. 50% to 66%

158. Which TWO pharmacokinetic processes are primarily responsible for determining the speed of onset and magnitude of drug effect?

    A. Absorption

    B. Distribution

    C. Metabolism

    D. Excretion

Match the following brain structures with their appropriate function:

159. Nucleus accumbens

160. Ventral tegmental area

161. Hippocampus

162. Medial prefrontal cortex

    A. Involved in memory formation

    B. Implicated in self-monitoring and self-evaluation of emotion

    C. Key structure in the mesolimbic reward circuit

163. Which of the following describes the mechanism of tricyclic antidepressants?

    A. They prevent the inactivation of biogenic amines.

    B. They block the reuptake of serotonin and norepinephrine to the presynaptic neuron.

    C. They block the reuptake of serotonin and norepinephrine to the postsynaptic neuron.

    D. They enhance the release of biogenic amines.

164. How often should fasting glucose and lipids be monitored after a pediatric patient has had 3 months of treatment with an antipsychotic?

    A. Every 3 months

    B. Every 6 months

    C. Every 12 months

    D. Not indicated if normal levels at 3 months

165. All the following are often a standard part of the assessment of a child that should be available before starting pharmacotherapy EXCEPT:

    A. ECG

    B. Height

    C. Body Mass Index

    D. Weight

    E. Vital signs

166. Youths under the age of 18 years are generally deemed not legally competent to make medical decisions; however, obtaining their agreement for treatment is often warranted. What is this usually called?

A. Consent

B. Assent

C. Coercion

D. Self-determination

167. Tic severity peaks in what decade of life?

A. First decade

B. Second decade

C. Third decade

D. Fourth decade

168. Sertraline has FDA approval for what disorder in children and adolescents?

A. Major depressive disorder

B. Generalized anxiety disorder

C. Obsessive-compulsive disorder

D. Posttraumatic stress disorder

169. Which of the following can act as partners in cytochrome P450 inhibition?

A. P-glycoprotein and glucuronic acid

B. CY1A2 and CY3A4

C. CY1A2 and P-glycoprotein

D. CY3A4 and P-glycoprotein

170. A teenager has stable levels of lithium and then starts taking ibuprofen for menstrual cramps. The increased lithium levels are the result of what type of interaction?

A. Pharmacogenetic reaction

B. Pharmacodynamic reaction

C. Pharmacokinetic reaction

D. None of the above

171. Which agent appears to be associated with the most rapid weight gain in antipsychotic-naïve youths?

A. Quetiapine

B. Olanzapine

C. Risperidone

D. Aripiprazole

172. All the following have FDA-approved uses for anxiety in children EXCEPT:

A. Fluvoxamine

B. Sertraline

C. Venlafaxine

D. Fluoxetine

173. Dysfunction of which interneurons in the associative and sensorimotor regions of the basal ganglia may underlie the emergence of tics and other forms of disinhibited behavior characterizing Tourette's symptomatology?

A. Serotonin

B. Norepinephrine

C. Glutamate

D. GABA

For questions 174 to 177, consider a clinical instrument with 85% sensitivity and 70% specificity that is used on a population with a 40% rate of the disorder being screened for.

174. What percentage of the total population would the clinical instrument correctly identify as having the disorder?

A. 8%

B. 26%

C. 34%

D. 46%

175. What percentage of the total population would the clinical instrument correctly identify as NOT having the disorder?

A. 6%

B. 18%

C. 34%

D. 42%

176. What percentage of the total population would the clinical instrument incorrectly identify as being without the disorder when they actually do have the disorder?

A. 1%

B. 6%

C. 12%

D. 18%

177. What percentage of the total population would the clinical instrument incorrectly identify as having the disorder when they actually do not have it?

   A. 12%

   B. 15%

   C. 18%

   D. 27%

178. Where is melatonin endogenously produced?

   A. Hypothalamus

   B. Basal ganglia

   C. Mammillary bodies

   D. Pineal gland

179. What is another name for St. John's wort?

   A. Kava

   B. Valerian

   C. Sarsaparilla

   D. Hypericum

   E. Rose hips

Match the following terms with their definitions:

180. Diffusion tensor imaging (DTI)

181. Fractional anisotropy (FA)

182. Apparent diffusion coefficient (ADC)

183. Resting-state functional connectivity

   A. An indicator of the magnitude of diffusion of water within the tissue, with lower values indicative of greater white matter organization

   B. A measure of the diffusion and directional selectivity of the random motion of water molecules within brain tissue

   C. A measure of the spontaneous, slow-wave fluctuations in blood oxygen level-dependent (BOLD) signal that are observed at rest and the interregional correlations of these temporal patterns

   D. Used to assess the integrity of white matter tracts in the brain

184. In most clinical trials, how many primary research hypotheses can be addressed?

   A. 1

   B. 3

   C. 5

   D. 9

185. This landmark legislation was a watershed accomplishment in the area of pediatric pharmacology research and essentially codified in statute the FDA's previously adopted regulation (the Pediatric Rule of 1998) mandating pediatric assessments for certain drug and biological applications.

   A. Pediatric Research Equity Act (PREA) of 2003

   B. Pediatric Use subsection under the Precautions section of labeling in 1979

   C. Food and Drug Administration Modernization Act (FDAMA) of 1997

   D. Food and Drug Administration Amendments Act (FDAAA) of 2007

   E. Best Pharmaceuticals for Children Act of 2001

186. The presence of major depressive disorder (MDD) in youths with which associated factor significantly elevates the risk for completed suicide?

   A. Parental depression

   B. Failing academic performance

   C. Antisocial peer group

   D. Substance abuse

187. The United States accounts for what percentage of worldwide consumption of stimulants?

   A. 10%

   B. 30%

   C. 55%

   D. 80%

188. Fetal hydantoin syndrome can occur from prenatal exposure to:

   A. Phenytoin

   B. Valproic acid

   C. Carbamazepine

   D. All of the above

189. **What is a major difference between childhood-onset and adult-onset obsessive-compulsive disorder (OCD)?**

    A. In children, compulsions often precede obsessions.

    B. In adults, compulsions are more often sensory in nature.

    C. Children have more insight into their symptoms.

    D. The majority of children undergo a developmental phase of OCD.

    E. Children have a better treatment response.

190. **The Preschool ADHD Treatment Study (PATS) revealed that the effect size of preschoolers with ADHD treated with methylphenidate was:**

    A. Equivalent to the effect size in older children treated with methylphenidate

    B. Greater than the effect size in older children treated with methylphenidate

    C. Less than the effect size in older children treated with methylphenidate

    D. Equivalent to the effect size of placebo treatment

191. **What term describes the common, but erroneous, belief held by many study subjects that their personal best interests will be served by research participation because the investigators are health-care professionals who in general must be committed to good patient care?**

    A. Therapeutic conflict of interest

    B. Therapeutic determinism

    C. Therapeutic denial

    D. Therapeutic misconception

192. **Benzodiazepines bind primarily to which receptor?**

    A. $GABA_A$ receptors

    B. $GABA_B$ receptors

    C. $GABA_C$ receptors

    D. None of the above

193. **Melatonin has which of the following effects?**

    A. Chronobiotic

    B. Neuroleptic

    C. Hypnotic

    D. Stimulant

    E. A and C

194. **The prevalence of specific phobia in children and adolescents appears to be highest in what age group?**

    A. 2 to 4

    B. 5 to 8

    C. 10 to 13

    D. 14 to 17

195. **A patient with significant liver impairment is being treated for anxiety. You are consulted on the case and examine his medication list. Which of the following agents would likely elicit the most concern?**

    A. Lorazepam

    B. Temazepam

    C. Diazepam

    D. Oxazepam

196. **What is one of the mechanisms of action of stimulants?**

    A. Reuptake blockade of catecholamines into presynaptic neurons, thereby preventing their degradation by tyrosine hydroxylase

    B. Reuptake blockade of catecholamines into presynaptic neurons, thereby preventing their degradation by monoamine oxidase

    C. Inhibition of monoamine oxidase degradation of catecholamines

    D. Increased monoamine oxidase synthesis

197. **Which is the only non-pharmacological treatment shown to improve neurocognitive deficits in early-onset schizophrenia spectrum disorders (EOSS)?**

    A. Cognitive behavioral therapy

    B. Cognitive remediation therapy

    C. Mentalization-based therapy

    D. Psychoanalysis

198. **Which TWO of the following medications are excreted unchanged from the body?**

    A. Risperidone

    B. Lithium

    C. Gabapentin

    D. Imipramine

199. Women who take lithium during the first trimester should have which of the following procedures between 18 and 20 weeks of gestation?

    A. Cardiac ultrasonography

    B. Maternal serum alpha-fetoprotein levels

    C. Sonography to screen for neural tube defects

    D. All of the above

200. Which of the following statements is true?

    A. The affinity of clonidine for alpha-2b and alpha-2c is greater than its affinity for alpha-2a.

    B. Guanfacine is 10 times less potent than clonidine in reducing presynaptic norepinephrine release.

    C. The affinity of guanfacine for alpha-2b and alpha-2c is greater than its affinity for alpha-2a.

    D. Guanfacine binds with moderate affinity to alpha-1 receptors.

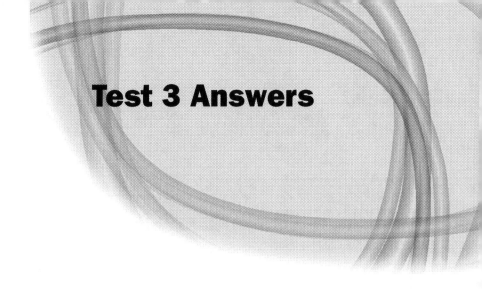

Test 3 Answers

1. Answer: D

For a full antagonist, approximately 60% to 75% dopamine receptor occupancy is needed for antipsychotic efficacy. For a partial agonist, receptor occupancy is not equivalent to blockade and a higher degree of occupancy (80% to 85%) is required to achieve the same level of blockade. (Chap. 23)

2. Answer: C

Trazodone, because of its alpha-adrenergic antagonism, can also cause orthostatic hypotension; it also has moderate antihistaminergic properties but has very little anticholinergic activity. (Chap. 21)

3. Answer: D

Avoiding milk products, chocolate, and caffeinated beverages is an important component in the maintenance treatment of chronic pediatric constipation. (Chap. 48)

4. Answer: E

Rett's disorder has been diagnosed almost exclusively in females. (Chap. 38)

5. Answer: C

Growing evidence indicates that untreated symptoms in pregnancy may lead to adverse medical outcomes, such as placental abruption as a reported consequence of maternal panic disorder. (Chap. 44)

6. Answer: D

Beneficence retains a virtuous hint of paternalism, in that the term captures the clinician's obligation to do and seek good for the patient. (Chap. 52)

7. Answer: D

Children are at risk for more severe illness. They do not appear at risk for increased rates of dysthymia. Childhood psychotic disorder is also associated with a family history of bipolar disorder and psychotic depression and an increased risk for resistance to antidepressant monotherapy. (Chap. 32)

8. Answer: A

Psychoeducation of the child, parents, and caregivers should be the first step. (Chap. 39)

9. Answer: C

Lithium was no different from placebo in reducing the severity of affective symptoms but it helped, statistically, reduce positive urine screens. (Chap. 41)

10. Answer: D

Modafinil is structurally and pharmacologically different than other agents approved for ADHD. In a 9-week, randomized, double-blind placebo-controlled trial, it was shown to have an effect size of 0.69. Given the number of pharmacotherapy options for ADHD and the rare occurrence of rash on modafinil, it was not FDA-approved. (It can still be prescribed off-label judiciously, with risks and benefits weighed.) (Chap. 31)

11. Answer: C

Valproate increases levels of lamotrigine. (Chap. 22)

12. Answer: C

The most common side effects of pregabalin are somnolence and dizziness. Other side effects include small weight gain, dry mouth, euphoria, incoordination, flatulence, and difficulty concentrating. (Chap. 24)

13. Answer: D

SLITRK1 contributes to the development of cortico-striatal-thalamic-cortical circuits. (Chap. 12)

14. Answer: B

Amnesia usually improves during the first few months after ECT, but some patients may have permanent memory loss for events that occurred before and close to the time of treatment. (Chap. 26)

15. Answer: D

In general, it takes five times the half-life of a drug for both steady state and elimination. (Chap. 23)

16. Answer: B

Diabetes insipidus due to lithium treatment is reversible if the medication is discontinued. (Chap. 22)

17. Answer: A and C

Fat stores and water distribution in the body determine the volume of distribution. For example, the proportion of body fat affects the volume of distribution of highly lipophilic drugs, including most neuroleptics and antidepressants. (Chap. 3)

18. Answer: C

Treatment of parental depression improves the risk of onset of childhood depression. (Chap. 32)

19. Answer: D

The rate of antipsychotic prescribing, overwhelmingly atypical agents by 2002, increased 6-fold. Most prescriptions were for disruptive behavior disorders, followed by mood disorders, pervasive developmental disorders, or intellectual disability, with psychotic disorders being the least common. (Chap. 49)

20. Answer: D

The rate of comorbid psychiatric disorders in adolescents with substance use disorders is 75% to 85%. The disorders with the highest prevalence are conduct disorder, ADHD, and mood disorders. (Chap. 41)

21. Answer: C

Incarcerated individuals have a two- to four-fold higher rate of epilepsy, but a correlation between criminal acts and seizure activity has not been demonstrated. Aggression during the interictal period is in response to social context (i.e., it is purposeful), and during the ictal or postictal period it is nondirected and unintentional. (Chap. 47)

22. Answer: C

The anxiety appears to increase the adherence. Children with bipolar disorder who also have anxiety are more likely to exhibit manic symptoms at an earlier age and have a higher likelihood of hospitalization and a poorer outcome. (Chap. 33)

23–26. Answers

23-B, 24-C, 25-A, 26-D. (Chap. 28)

27. Answer: A

Randomized clinical trials have been broadly categorized as having either a pragmatic or explanatory approach. (Chap. 29)

28. Answer: C

A polar drug that is non-lipid-soluble and has a large molecular size is more difficult to absorb. (Chap. 3)

29. Answer: C

Desmopressin acetate is an arginine vasopressin (AVP) analogue, and the response is dose-dependent. (Chap. 48)

30. Answer: A

The ratio changes to a 2-to-1 female-to-male preponderance by adolescence, as it is in adulthood. (Chap. 9)

31. Answer: D

Dopaminergic neurons projecting from the hypothalamus to the pituitary gland are called the tuberoinfundibular projection. (Chap. 2)

32. Answer: A

An effect size of 0.3 is considered small. (Chap. 29)

33. Answer: B

The lateral fusiform gyrus is located in the ventral occipital temporal cortex and, due to its selective role in processing faces, has been called the "fusiform face area." (Chap. 14)

34. Answer: C

Liver enzyme testing should be considered in patients who have signs of fatty liver infiltration. (Chap. 23)

35. Answer: A and C

The hippocampus and amygdala compose the medial lobe. (Chap. 2)

36. Answer: C

Anecdotal evidence suggests stimulants may help with hyperactivity, impulsivity, and inattention, which can be found in childhood PTSD. (Chap. 39)

37. Answer: B

MAO-B accounts for 80% of the CNS monoamine oxidase. (Chap. 21)

38. Answer: B

There is a high prevalence of binge eating disorder or a loss of control over eating in overweight youths; eating disorders should be investigated. (Chap. 40)

39. Answer: B

Compared with adults, children are more likely to have mixed or rapid-cycling bipolar disorder. (Chap. 42)

40. Answer: A

Gingko biloba has been studied as a treatment for Alzheimer's disease and dementia with negative results. (Chap. 25)

41. Answer: B

Plasma half-life is also known as the elimination half-life, which describes the time required for the concentration of drug to decrease by 50%. (Chap. 3)

42. Answer: A

Significant hypoleptinemia occurs in acute anorexia nervosa, which usually triggers amenorrhea because the secretion of luteinizing and follicle-stimulating hormone depends on critical serum leptin thresholds. Consequently, hypoleptinemia could be considered a biological marker of anorexia nervosa. (Chap. 16)

43. Answer: E

There are several lines of research in pharmacogenomic testing of polymorphisms. (Chap. 20)

44. Answer: A

Buspirone has been shown to reduce SSRI-induced sexual dysfunction. (Chap. 24)

45. Answer: C

The half-life of citalopram in teenagers is 38.4 hours, compared to 44 hours in adults. (Chap. 20)

46. Answer: C

Carbamazepine does not have strong evidence for use as a first-line agent. Moreover, carbamazepine's numerous P450 drug interactions make its clinical use difficult. (Chap. 22)

47. Answer: D

The treatment approach will depend on a number of factors. Generally, CBT alone or combination treatment is recommended first, but all three would be acceptable. (Chap. 34)

48. Answer: A

Medications should be considered if the tics interfere with a child's life. This interference may take the form of impaired concentration due to the distraction of premonitory sensations, direct pain or injury from specific tics, disruption in school due to vocal tics, teasing due to highly noticeable tics, or reduced self-esteem due to social stigma. There is no evidence that medication improves the course or severity of Tourette's disorder, and parental concerns need to be addressed but this may involve psychoeducation. (Chap. 36)

49. Answer: A

Generally, one should consider treating mania first, since treatment of ADHD may exacerbate manic symptoms. (Chap. 27)

50–53. Answers

50-D; 51-B; 52-A, C; 53-A, C.

These are FDA-labeled indications. Physicians may use medications off-label. (Chap. 51)

54. Answer: A

Pharmacogenomics, used interchangeably with pharmacogenetics, refers to an area of research that employs genetic information for drug design and development. (Chap. 6)

55. Answer: D

Pregabalin is FDA-indicated as adjunctive therapy for partial-onset seizures, neuropathic pain, and post-herpetic neuralgia. (Chap. 22)

56. Answer: B

The class II, G-protein-coupled receptors represent the slow-acting class of receptors of the postsynaptic cell. (Chap. 2)

57. Answer: D

Anticholinergic effects of antihistamines include dry mouth and respiratory passages, cough, urinary retention, and dysuria. Other side effects of antihistamines include sedation, dizziness, tinnitus, lassitude, incoordination, fatigue, blurred vision, diplopia, euphoria, nervousness, insomnia, nausea, vomiting, constipation, diarrhea, and tremor. (Chap. 24)

58. Answer: E

Carbamazepine is both highly bioavailable and protein bound. (Chap. 22)

59. Answer: D

VNS has been proven effective in treating refractory epilepsy in children and adults and is being investigated in the treatment of adult depression and anxiety disorders. (Chap. 26)

60. Answer: C

The emergence of federally sponsored multi-site studies has played a significant role in the knowledge base of pediatric psychopharmacology. (Chap. 49)

61. Answer: D

The rate of smooth pursuit eye movement abnormalities is higher than what has been reported with adult-onset schizophrenia and is close to 80%. (Chap. 13)

62. Answer: D

The rate of responders in each treatment group can be determined by using a global measurement of improvement for each subject or selecting a priori a cutoff score on a continuous symptom scale. The rate of positive response in each group conveys clinically relevant and easily interpretable information about the effectiveness of treatment and can be used to compute the number needed to treat (NNT). (Chap. 50)

63. Answer: C

Methylphenidate has been found to be effective for the neurocognitive sequelae of childhood cancers. (Chap. 43)

64. Answer: C

Risperidone appears safe to use in seizure disorders. (Chap. 43)

65. Answer: E

Valproate is highly protein-bound and is metabolized in the liver. (Chap. 22)

66. Answer: B

CYP1A2 and CYP2E1 levels are higher in males than females, and activities of CYP2B6, CYP3A4, and potentially CYP2D6 are greater in females. (Chap. 4)

67. Answer: B

Selective mutism usually has its onset before the age of 5 and typically occurs in the age range of 2 to 4. (Chap. 34)

68. Answer: C

30% to 50% of substance-use disorders begin in childhood or adolescence. (Chap. 41)

69. Answer: D

The absence of variation (and extreme scores) on a clinical instrument may signal a tendency of the parent to view the child in overly positive or negative terms. (Chap. 28)

70. Answer: B

After clinical trials are completed, depending on the results, the company will submit a New Drug Application. (Chap. 51)

71. Answer: A

One meta-analytic study in mostly adult patients found the effect size of SSRIs in GAD to be 0.36. (Chap. 24)

72. Answer: C

There appears to be less risk of tardive dyskinesia with atypical antipsychotics. (Chap. 36)

73. Answer: A

This question is intended to indicate the significant effectiveness of ECT treatment for certain psychiatric illnesses. (Chap. 26)

74. Answer: E

An asymptomatic drop in blood pressure of 10% can occur but is uncommon rather than common. Nervousness, agitation, headache, nightmares, frequent waking, weight gain, and nausea and vomiting are reported but less frequently so. Hypotension and bradycardia have also been observed, but large-scale trials suggest that these problems rarely prompt discontinuation. (Chap. 19)

75. Answer: D

Oxcarbazepine is an analogue of carbamazepine. (Chap. 22)

76. Answer: C

TCAs have not been shown to be superior to placebo. Moreover, the side-effect profile of TCAs further weakens the indication of this class of medication to treat pediatric depression. (Chap. 32)

77. Answer: B

Clomipramine is FDA-approved for OCD in children older than 10 years. (Chap. 21)

78. Answer: D

Phase III trials are randomized controlled trials that test hypotheses and efficacy in a conclusive way. (Chap. 50)

79. Answer: C

The muscle relaxant is administered for ECT when the patient is well sedated; otherwise, the patient would be paralyzed but conscious. (Chap. 26)

80. Answer: C

All serotonin receptors are G-protein-coupled receptors except $5HT_3$, which is an ionic receptor. (Chap. 2)

81. Answer: D

All the compounds, as well as bethanechol, are agonists of muscarinic receptors. (Chap. 2)

82. Answer: B

Alpha-2 agonists mimic NE actions at post-synaptic alpha-2A receptors in the PFC. (Chap. 11)

83. Answer: D

The dorsal PFC and the lateral PFC use representational knowledge (working memory) to guide movement and attention. (Chap. 11)

84. Answer: B

For SSRIs in general, but especially for long-acting fluoxetine, 2 to 5 drug-free weeks are required to prevent elevated risks of serotonin syndrome. (Chap. 21)

85. Answer: B

The prevalence of elimination disorders in school-age children is 2% to 7%. (Chap. 48)

86. Answer: A

ADHD is the most commonly presenting juvenile psychiatric disorder. (Chap. 31)

87. Answer: A

Glutamatergic neurons and NMDA receptors in the hippocampus are important for long-term potentiation. (Chap. 2)

88. Answer: B

The most prevalent of childhood disorders in epidemiological studies is anxiety disorder, with 6% to 20% of children affected. ADHD more commonly comes to professional attention because of its disruptive nature. (Chap. 34)

89. Answer: D

Quetiapine has one randomized controlled trial showing no effect and another randomized trial comparing it against divalproex sodium showing benefit for both. Olanzapine was found to be helpful in a population of children with autistic spectrum diagnoses. Iloperidone may or may not be useful, but there are no data. Clozapine has adult controlled data showing usefulness for aggression and suicidality. (Chap. 47)

90. Answer: D

The same study also indicated that non-Caucasians had an increased risk of tardive dyskinesia upon exposure to antipsychotics. (Chap. 37)

91. Answer: B

In a crossover design the subjects are given all the treatments sequentially in random order. A disadvantage is that there can be carryover effects from one treatment to another. Subjects who receive active treatment first often show greater benefit than those who receive active treatment after placebo. (Chap. 50)

92. Answer: C

Non-adrenergic–located alpha-2 receptors inhibit the release of several neurotransmitters, including dopamine and glutamate. This is consistent with the general calming effects of alpha-2 agonists. (Chap. 19)

93. Answer: B

Besides the gonadal hormones, low leptin levels play a role in bone density loss through activation of the hypothalamus-pituitary axis, leading to hypercortisolism. Hypoleptinemia may also inhibit bone reabsorption. (Chap. 40)

94. Answer: C

Many of the disorder association and pharmacogenetic studies have examined a functional VNTR (variable number tandem repeats) polymorphism in the promoter region of the serotonin transporter gene (HTT), the so-called 5-HTTLPR. The transporter is a critical component of the serotonergic system and is the principal site of action of the widely prescribed SSRIs. (Chap. 6)

95. Answer: C

For mild and moderate cases, CBT is recommended as a first-line treatment. For more severe cases, combination treatment is recommended. (Chap. 35)

96. Answer: B

NMDA is a subclass of a glutamate receptor. (Chap. 38)

97. Answer: B

Olanzapine was rated second in helpfulness in treating behaviors of physical aggression and destruction of property. (Chap. 42)

98. Answer: D

Interactions for fluvoxamine run from the weaker 2D6 to the significant 1A2. The latter's substrates include acetaminophen, caffeine, propranolol, and theophylline; fluvoxamine slows their metabolism. (Chap. 20)

99. Answer: C

EPS symptoms in youths present more commonly, so clinicians should proactively monitor for cogwheeling, drooling, and reduced arm swing, particularly when doses are being increased. (Chap. 37)

100. Answer: D

The question highlights the presence of several tools specifically intended for children with intellectual disability. (Chap. 42)

101. Answer: D

The listed conditions are considered high risk for ECT, but there are no absolute contraindications for ECT. (Chap. 26)

102. Answer: B

Preclinical testing is done with animals. At least two animal species are exposed to a wide range of doses of the drug for varying durations, and assessments include observation for abnormal signs, routine measurements (laboratory parameters, vital signs, electrocardiograms), and both gross anatomical and histopathological evaluation. Plasma is sampled for concentrations of parent drug and metabolites to estimate pharmacokinetic parameters and to *attempt to discover plasma concentration–adverse effect relationships. (Chap. 51)*

103. Answer: C

Although prolactin levels are not tightly correlated with sexual dysfunction, hyperprolactinemia can result in sexual side effects, such as amenorrhea or oligomenor-rhea, erectile dysfunction, decreased libido, hirsutism, and breast symptoms, such as enlargement, engorgement, pain, or galactorrhea. (Chap. 23)

104. Answer: C

A serious rash while on lamotrigine, which can occur in up to 1% of patients, requires hospitalization and discontinuation of treatment. (Chap. 22)

105. Answer: D

If whistle blowing occurs unethically or is resorted to with undue haste, reputations can be sullied by inaccurate or malicious accusations. (Chap. 53)

106. Answer: A

Atomoxetine is a specific norepinephrine reuptake inhibitor. (Chap. 31)

107. Answer: C

Two studies (Lavigne et al., 1998; Cesena et al., 2002) indicate there is a high risk for preschool children with disruptive behavior disorders to develop an additional psychiatric disorder. (Chap. 45)

108. Answer: E

All of the above statements are true. One erroneous conclusion at times drawn from the results is that stimulants were not effective; instead, it shows that regardless of which arm you were assigned to **initially***, the later outcomes were similar. Many patients originally assigned to medications stopped stimulants; some of those who had received behavioral treatment started using stimulants; and all subjects were transferred to community care as usual after the initial 18 months, and this care had already been shown to be less effective than the research-based academic center care. (Chap. 18)*

109. Answer: C

Rituals during meals, eating separately from the family, drinking excessive or minimal amounts of liquid, increased physical activity, and wearing loosely fitting clothes might be signs of an eating disorder. (Chap. 40)

110. Answer: D

Children with EOSS shift from multimodal hallucinations to predominantly auditory hallucinations during adolescence. (Chap. 37)

111. Answer: B

Clinical effect is seen as early as 30 minutes after administration. (Chap. 18)

112. Answer: A

MAO-B is important in dopamine metabolism. (Chap. 15)

113. Answer: A

Desipramine and nortriptyline selectively block the norepinephrine transporter. (Chap. 2)

114. Answer: C

The cause is unknown in approximately 70% of cases of major birth defects. (Chap. 44)

115. Answer: E

The goal of FFT-A is to reduce symptoms by decreasing levels of expressed emotion from family members and improving family problem-solving and communication skills. (Chap. 33)

116. Answer: C

Clonidine is available as a transdermal patch, which avoids the need for repeat dosing and may help reduce the sedation and dry mouth found with oral delivery. The patch is changed every 7 days (although some suggest 5 or 6 days is more appropriate). It is available as 0.1 mg, 0.2 mg, or 0.3 mg. (Chap. 36)

117. Answer: C

Projections from the nucleus accumbens innervate brain structures important for motor control, and prelimbic inputs are critical to mediating drug seeking in the addicted animal. (Chap. 17)

118. Answer: C

By some definitions, manic symptoms occur for greater than 4 hours daily in ultradian cycling. (Chap. 33)

119. Answer: C

Guanfacine is a specific alpha-2a agonist; clonidine non-specifically targets alpha 2a, 2b, and 2c. (Chap. 19)

120. Answer: C

94.9% of visits for ADHD to family practitioners resulted in a prescription compared to 75.4% of visits to pediatricians and 74.2% of visits to psychiatrists. (Chap. 49)

121. Answer: C

Unless benzodiazepines are taken in combination with other drugs, such as ethanol, they do not appear to cause respiratory depression even at relatively high doses. (Chap. 24)

122. Answer: A

However, increased slow-wave sleep may increase the risk of partial arousal parasomnias, such as sleepwalking, in susceptible individuals. (Chap. 46)

123. Answer: D

Bupropion is not recommended for patients with bulimia or any other metabolic instability, such as uncontrolled diabetes, due to the risk of seizures. (Chap. 21)

124. Answer: D

In these studies, imipramine was found to be effective in 10% to 60% of typically developing children, but relapse rates following treatment were more than 90%. (Chap. 42)

125. Answer: A

Metformin, topiramate, amantadine, and orlistat have been used to treat pediatric obesity in youths taking antipsychotics. Use of these agents has not been adopted as standard clinical care, although data may increasingly emerge to suggest which subpopulations may benefit from adjunctive medication to prevent or reduce weight gain. (Chap. 23)

126. Answer: D

Abuse potential is a black box warning for stimulants. For euphoric effects they must be insufflated typically or used intravenously; there is a greater risk with immediate-release formulations that can be crushed. (Chap. 31)

127. Answer: B

The CDRS-Revised is clinician-administered. In clinical trials a clinician-administered scale is generally preferred. (Chap. 50)

128. Answer: A

Medication should be continued for 6 to 12 months after stabilization; the medication should be withdrawn slowly over several months. (Chap. 35)

129. Answer: D

Currently all stimulants used to treat ADHD and atomoxetine carry language to alert prescribers and consumers of a potential association between certain drugs used to treat ADHD (i.e., stimulants and atomoxetine) and sudden cardiovascular death in children with structural cardiac defects or a family history of such illness. (Chap. 51)

130. Answer: B

A strong alliance in pharmacotherapy appears linked to positive clinical outcomes. (Chap. 30)

131. Answer: D

Duloxetine is also FDA-approved for major depressive disorder and generalized anxiety disorder. (Chap. 21)

132. Answer: D

Currently, no medications are approved for use as hypnotics in children by the FDA. (Chap. 46)

133. Answer: A

The increase in surface area is not matched by a corresponding increase in thickness; although the surface area of the human cortex is 1000-fold larger than that of a mouse, it is only three-fold thicker. (Chap. 1)

134. Answer: B

Developmental delay does not raise suspicion for bipolar disorder, whereas episodic mood lability, early-onset depression, and drug-induced mania do; drug-induced mania should not, however, be overly weighted in making the diagnosis, since activation is common in children. The presence of psychosis and episodic aggressive behavior also raises suspicion of bipolar disorder. (Chap. 33)

135. Answer: A

Although youths who abuse substances are unlikely to abuse stimulants, and adult studies show that stimulants do not appear to increase craving, it is best to use other agents as first-line treatment. If stimulants are used, those with low abuse potential should be considered, such as lisdexamfetamine or OROS methylphenidate. (Chap. 41)

136. Answer: D

Olanzapine also increases alanine aminotransferase, aspartate aminotransferase, and insulin levels. (Chap. 37)

137. Answer: B

Rates of the disorder show a relatively marked decline from childhood to adolescence. (Chap. 10)

138. Answer: B

The number of indicated sessions of ECT in children and adolescents is likely similar to adults. However, the total number of ECT sessions should be based on treatment response and not guided by a predetermined number. (Chap. 26)

139. Answer: A

As of this publication, there is only one small RCT in youths ages 6 to 12 with major depression reporting a significant reduction in depressive symptoms. Studies in adults with major depression also show benefit. (Chap. 25)

140. Answer: A

There is no correction for placebo in open-label trials, so subsequent trials almost invariably show a smaller benefit. (Chap. 50)

141. Answer: C

85% of ideal body weight corresponds to a BMI of 10%. (Chap. 16)

142. Answer: C

In this cohort of preschool children, frequent hyperactivity was related specifically to deficits of visuospatial organization. (Chap. 15)

143. Answer: A

25 to 50 mg with a repeat dose as indicated is a reasonable dose. (Chap. 43)

144. Answer: B

The 14-week study included 158 children and adolescents at 19 sites and was funded by Autism Speaks and industry. The preliminary results were published in a press release (Autism Speaks, 2009). (Chap. 38)

145. Answer: B

The glutamate transporter gene SLCL1A1 is the only one to have been consistently replicated for OCD. Currently, a large international study using genome-wide association, which offers more power to identify risk genes by genotyping hundreds of thousands of markers across all chromosomes, is being undertaken. (Chap. 11)

146. Answer: D

Cytochrome P450 enzymes are a superfamily of heme-containing enzymes. (Chap. 4)

147. Answer: B

From the limited evidence, family-based interventions work best for children and adolescents with anorexia nervosa; if there is a high degree of conflict, sessions with the child and parents separately might be indicated. (Chap. 40)

148. Answer: B

There is no statistically significant increase in suicidal thinking on SSRIs in pooled data from pediatric OCD trials. The effect appears greater in depression studies. (Chap. 35)

149. Answer: D

Mirtazapine co-administration with alcohol and benzodiazepines can lead to synergistic effects on motor and cognitive performance. (Chap. 21)

150. Answer: C

Duloxetine is FDA-approved in adults for diabetic neuropathy and fibromyalgia. The data for its use in adolescent major depression and chronic pain are limited to case reports. (Chap. 43)

151. Answer: A

Stimulation of alpha-2 receptors enhances functioning in the prefrontal cortex. Conversely, stimulation of beta and alpha-1 receptors reduces functioning in the prefrontal cortex. (Chap. 11)

152. Answer: C

Standard practice suggests that blood pressure and pulse be obtained prior to starting treatment and monitored during treatment. A physical exam and a cardiac history are also indicated. An ECG might be indicated if the personal or family history suggests cardiac concerns of note. (Chap. 19)

153. Answer: D

Harm obsessions are the most common obsessions in children; these include fear of death or fear of illness befalling the self or a loved one. (Chap. 35)

154. Answer: B

Lithium has been found useful in two trials and not useful in two others. (Chap. 47)

155. Answer: B

The SSRIs may be more effective than other agents for avoidance and numbing. (Chap. 39)

156. Answer: B

The temporal lobe, in addition to the prefrontal cortex, has also been linked to aggressive behavior. (Chap. 15)

157. Answer: D

Retrospective studies of adults with bipolar disorder, not the most reliable type of data, indicate that up to two-thirds of patients report onset before 19 years of age. (Chap. 33)

158. Answer: A and B

Absorption and distribution of a drug primarily determine the speed of onset and magnitude of effect. (Chap. 3)

159–162. Answers

159-C, 160-C, 161-A, 162-B.

Memory formation involves the hippocampus; self-monitoring involves the medial prefrontal cortex; and the nucleus accumbens and the ventral tegmental area are involved in the mesolimbic reward circuit. (Chap. 8)

163. Answer: B

Initially blocking of reuptake leads to increased concentrations of serotonin and norepinephrine, but the subsequent net effect is increased serotonergic and noradrenergic neurotransmission. (Chap. 21)

164. Answer: C

Fasting glucose and lipids should be monitored at baseline, after 3 months of treatment, and at least annually thereafter. (Chap. 37)

165. Answer: A

ECG is not a standard part of the assessment before starting pharmacotherapy. A physical exam in the year prior to treatment should have been performed and height, weight, vital signs, and BMI would generally be available to and/ or performed by the prescribing clinician. (Chap. 27)

166. Answer: B

Assent, or agreement, to the plan of care has several moral, ethical, and therapeutic benefits. (Chap. 52)

167. Answer: B

Tics peak in severity between the ages of 10 to 12. (Chap. 12)

168. Answer: C

Sertraline has FDA approval for OCD in children ages 6 to 17. In adults, FDA approval is for MDD, OCD, PTSD, social anxiety disorder, panic disorder, and premenstrual dysphoric disorder. (Chap. 20)

169. Answer: D

Some drugs are both P-gp and CY3A4 inhibitors. P-gp can act as a gatekeeper to a drug's contact with CYP enzymes in the intestine, preventing entry. As the drug enters through the intestine it is inhibited by CY3A4. Double inhibitors (such as erythromycin) are more likely to cause clinically significant interactions. (Chap. 4)

170. Answer: C

This is a pharmacokinetic reaction (a non-cytochrome-mediated one); the ibuprofen decreases the renal clearance of lithium. (Chap. 4)

171. Answer: B

Olanzapine is associated with the most total weight gain and most rapid weight gain. (Chap. 23)

172. Answer: C

Venlafaxine has shown positive results but does not have FDA approval; one can use it off-label, although data suggest that venlafaxine has higher rates of induced suicidal thinking than other similar agents. (Chap. 34)

173. Answer: D

Fast-spiking GABA-ergic interneuron dysfunction may underlie emergence of tics and other related symptoms. (Chap. 12)

174. Answer: C

The calculation for the sensitivity is 85% × 40%. (Chap. 28)

175. Answer: D

The calculation involves multiplying the given specificity, which is 70% by 60%—that is, the true percentage of the population not having the disorder. (Chap. 28)

176. Answer: B

The false-negative rate is determined by the calculation of 15% (100% of the population subtracted by the sensitivity of 85%) times the rate of the disorder (40%). (Chap. 28)

177. Answer: C

The false-positive rate is determined by the calculation of 30% (100% of the population subtracted by the given specificity of 70%) times the percentage of the population who do NOT have the disorder (60%). (Chap. 28)

178. Answer: D

Melatonin (N-acetyl-5-methoxytryptamine) is produced in the pineal gland. (Chap. 24)

179. Answer: D

St. John's wort is also known as Hypericum perforatum or hypericum. (Chap. 25)

180–183. Answers

180-D, 181-B, 182-A, 183-C. (Chap. 9)

184. Answer: A

In most clinical trials only one primary research hypothesis can be addressed. Secondary hypotheses can be examined, but sub-analyses often do not have the statistical power needed. (Chap. 50)

185. Answer: A

The PREA of 2003 gave the FDA statutory authority to require pediatric studies. The PREA requirements were also made retroactive to April 1, 1999. As a result, all drug and biological applications approved on April 1, 1999, or thereafter were required to submit to the FDA a Pediatric Plan that outlines the studies that the sponsor plans to conduct or request a waiver or deferral of the pediatric study requirements. (Chap. 51)

186. Answer: D

Substance abuse worsens the prognosis of depression and increases the risk of completed suicide. (Chap. 32)

187. Answer: D

The United States accounts for 80% of worldwide consumption of stimulants. (Chap. 18)

188. Answer: D

Fetal hydantoin syndrome consisting of facial dimorphism, nail dysplasia, digital hypoplasia, cleft lip and palate, cardiac defects, and cognitive abnormalities can occur with prenatal exposure to phenytoin as well as other anticonvulsants. (Chap. 44)

189. Answer: A

Children often have compulsions that precede their obsessions. Children have less insight into their symptoms and their symptoms are more frequently sensory in nature. Children have a less robust treatment response. Children find security in rituals and sameness, but frank OCD is not developmentally normal. (Chap. 11)

190. Answer: C

Although significantly superior to placebo, the effect size of stimulants for ADHD in PATS is lower than that reported in older children. (Chap. 45)

191. Answer: D

Therapeutic misconception in research refers to the notion that subjects believe their personal best interests will be served, even though the research objectives are paramount. This happens even when informed consent is thorough. (Chap. 52)

192. Answer: A

Benzodiazepines bind primarily to type 1 and type 2 GABA$_A$ receptors. (Chap. 24)

193. Answer: E

Depending on the dose and time of administration, melatonin can shift the circadian sleep–wake cycle (chronobiotic) and be slightly sedating (mild hypnotic). (Chap. 46)

194. Answer: C

The highest prevalence of specific phobia in childhood occurs between 10 and 13 years old. (Chap. 10)

195. Answer: C

Diazepam undergoes phase I oxidation and dealkylation and phase II conjugation in the liver, whereas lorazepam, oxazepam, and temazepam undergo phase II only and are therefore better tolerated. Diazepam remains an option, but greater consideration is warranted. (Chap. 24)

196. Answer: B

Stimulants block reuptake of catecholamines into presynaptic neurons, thereby preventing their degradation by monoamine oxidase. (Chap. 31)

197. Answer: B

There has been some evidence of limited improvement in cognitive flexibility, but other improvements in cognition have not been seen. (Chap. 37)

198. Answer: B and C

Gabapentin and lithium are excreted unchanged from the body. (Chap. 3)

199. Answer: A

Cardiac ultrasonography to examine the fetal heart. Women exposed to anticonvulsants (valproic acid and carbamazepine among others) during pregnancy should be screened for serum alpha-fetoprotein levels, screened for neural tube defects by sonography, and have an amniocentesis to evaluate alpha-fetoprotein levels. (Chap. 44)

200. Answer: B

Guanfacine is 10 times less potent than clonidine in reducing presynaptic norepinephrine release in the locus coeruleus (LC) or inhibiting LC firing. The other answer options are true statements if phrased oppositely. (Chap. 19)

Test 4 Questions

1. Which of the following medications increases triglycerides?

   A. Aripiprazole

   B. Olanzapine

   C. Quetiapine

   D. B and C

2. In a clinical trial, statistical significance may not be clinically relevant. What can be used to demonstrate clinical significance?

   A. Chi-square test

   B. Effect size

   C. Power

   D. Sensitivity

3. Which of the following statements is accurate regarding attention-deficit/hyperactivity disorder (ADHD) in adolescents?

   A. Adolescents with ADHD are less likely to smoke than ADHD-free peers.

   B. Adolescents with ADHD who are prescribed stimulants may be at higher risk for substance abuse than ADHD peers without treatment.

   C. Adolescents with ADHD are less likely to have a depressive disorder than ADHD-free peers.

   D. Adolescents with ADHD are at increased risk for substance use.

4. The dopamine hypotheses of Tourette's disorder encompass all the following EXCEPT:

   A. Excess of dopamine

   B. Increased sensitivity of D2 dopamine receptors

   C. Antipsychotics that preferentially block D2 receptors are effective

   D. Decreased sensitivity of D2 dopamine receptors

5. Which of the following is an antagonist to the 5-HT$_3$ receptor?

   A. Fluoxetine

   B. Ondansetron

   C. Scopolamine

   D. Bethanechol

6. In adults being treated for depression, the dose of EPA+DHA is at least 1 gram daily. What is the suggested dose for children?

   A. 25 mg of EPA and 10 mg of DHA

   B. 50 mg of EPA and 25 mg of DHA

   C. 400 mg of EPA and 200 mg of DHA

   D. 2200 mg of EPA and 1100 mg of DHA

7. Most controlled trials support the efficacy of which medication for the treatment of attention-deficit/hyperactivity disorder (ADHD) in youths?

   A. Fluoxetine

   B. Desipramine

   C. Methylphenidate

   D. B and C

8. Interpersonal and Social Rhythm Therapy (IPSRT) for adolescents with bipolar disorder focuses on which TWO triggers as potentially causing recurrence of mood episodes?

   A. Circadian rhythms

   B. Lack of social supports

   C. Increased expressed emotion in family members

   D. Problems in interpersonal relationships

9. What are fairly consistent findings in MRI morphometric measurements of the brain in OCD patients?

    A. Decrease in subcortical structures

    B. Increase in occipital volume

    C. Decrease in frontal cortex volume

    D. Increased fourth ventricular volume

10. Semi-starvation (or acute anorexia nervosa)-induced hypoleptinemia causes which of the following to occur?

    A. Amenorrhea

    B. Hyperactivity

    C. Weight loss

    D. A and B

11. In what decade of life is the primary onset of eating disorders?

    A. First

    B. Second

    C. Third

    D. Fourth

12. The Pediatric Rule of 1998 and the Pediatric Research Equity Act of 2003 required pediatric studies from a pharmaceutical sponsor whose submission for a new drug application contained which of the following?

    A. New ingredient, indication, dosage form, color, route of administration

    B. New ingredient, indication, dosage form, dosing regimen, route of administration

    C. New ingredient, indication, taste, dosing regimen, route of administration

    D. New ingredient, indication, dosage form, dosing regimen, fillers

13. In the clinically meaningful metric of effect size, a medium magnitude of effect is represented by which of the following decimals?

    A. 0.3

    B. 0.5

    C. 0.7

    D. 0.8

14. Which term describes how consistent a screening or diagnostic instrument is from one administration to another and from one rater to another?

    A. Reliability

    B. Validity

    C. Sensitivity

    D. Specificity

15. What do amphetamines do?

    A. Block reuptake of catecholamines into presynaptic neurons

    B. Cause retrograde release of catecholamines through the transporter

    C. Act on the vesicular storage of catecholamines

    D. All of the above

    E. None of the above

16. The DSM-IV diagnosis of dysthymic disorder (DD) in children requires the presence of depressed mood or irritability on most days for most of the day for at least what duration of time?

    A. 2 weeks

    B. 1 month

    C. 2 months

    D. 1 year

17. Which of the following monoamine oxidase inhibitors has selective irreversible inhibition of monoamine oxidase-B (MAO-B)?

    A. Phenelzine

    B. Selegiline

    C. Tranylcypromine

    D. Isocarboxazid

18. In a 4-year follow-up study of 86 patients with pre-pubertal-onset bipolar disorder, the presence of psychosis predicted which of the following?

    A. Increased risk of substance-use disorders

    B. Greater severity of depressive symptoms

    C. More frequent cycling

    D. Longer duration of mania or hypomania

19. What is one of the problems with "whistle blowing"?

    A. It costs money.

    B. It helps bring misdeeds to light.

    C. Whistle blowing is unethical.

    D. Reputations can be damaged if whistle blowing is conducted hastily.

20. Which of the following time frames corresponds best to a period in which the patient is in the maintenance phase of treatment for major depressive disorder (MDD)?

    A. 1 month

    B. 3 months

    C. 6 months

    D. 12 months

21. What happens in phase I drug metabolism?

    A. Cytochrome P450 enzymes reduce drugs to more readily excreted forms.

    B. Cytochrome P450 enzymes oxidize drugs to more readily excreted forms.

    C. Cytochrome P450 enzymes methylate drugs to more readily excreted forms.

    D. A sufyl group is added to reduce a drug's ability to react with other molecules.

22. Interventions to promote sleep hygiene include all of the following EXCEPT:

    A. Environmental

    B. Sleep–wake scheduling

    C. Bedtime routine

    D. Physiological

    E. Pharmacological

23. How many days does it take to achieve steady-state plasma levels of aripiprazole?

    A. 2 days

    B. 4 days

    C. 7 days

    D. 14 days

24. What is the first-line approach for the treatment of catatonia in pediatric patients?

    A. Electroconvulsive therapy

    B. Haloperidol

    C. Risperidone

    D. Lorazepam

25. Cognitive deficits associated with electroconvulsive therapy (ECT) are lower with which type of ECT?

    A. Unilateral

    B. Bilateral

    C. Equal deficits with both types

    D. None of the above

26. The clinical effect of immediate-release amphetamine and methylphenidate lasts approximately how long?

    A. 2 hours

    B. 4 hours

    C. 8 hours

    D. 12 hours

27. Which of the following is a recommended practice for discontinuing mirtazapine in patients?

    A. Prompt discontinuation over 1 to 2 days

    B. Decreasing the dose by 15 mg every 2 to 3 days

    C. Cross-tapering with fluoxetine

    D. Slow discontinuation over 1 to 2 months

28. Which country has the highest prevalence of two or more medications prescribed simultaneously to a young person?

    A. United States

    B. France

    C. Australia

    D. Italy

29. Which of the following is one of several reasonable research hypotheses for a clinical trial?

    A. What is the appropriate safe dosage to try?

    B. Is the treatment effective in reversing functional impairment?

    C. How should the medication be delivered—by mouth, intranasally, or intramuscularly?

    D. Can the medication be metabolized?

30. Which TWO pharmacokinetic processes are primarily responsible for terminating the action of the pharmacologic agent upon the body?

    A. Absorption

    B. Distribution

    C. Metabolism

    D. Excretion

31. Once a pharmaceutical company has done sufficient chemistry and manufacturing work to have a drug substance that is suitable for human testing and has completed sufficient preclinical studies, what happens next?

    A. Investigational New Drug (IND) application

    B. Phase 0 trial

    C. Phase 1 trial

    D. Animal testing

Match the following brain structures with the listed functions:

32. **Thalamus**

33. **Association cortex**

34. **Medial temporal lobe**

35. **Basal ganglia**

    A. Creates an internal representation of sensory information

    B. The gateway for all incoming sensory information to cortical processing

    C. Integrates multimodal sensory information for storage into and retrieval from memory, and attaches limbic valence to sensory information

    D. Integration of input from cortical areas

36. **What level of QTc prolongation is considered pathological?**

    A. >200 ms

    B. >300 ms

    C. >400 ms

    D. >500 ms

37. **Which of the following medications decreases rapid eye movement (REM) stage sleep?**

    A. SSRIs

    B. Opioids

    C. Lithium

    D. Corticosteroids

    E. All of the above

38. **Which of the following is most likely to occur upon abrupt discontinuation of clonidine?**

    A. Tachypnea

    B. Hypopnea

    C. Hypotension

    D. Angioedema

    E. Rash

39. **Which of the following compounds that blocks the NMDA receptor can induce psychotic symptoms?**

    A. Ketamine

    B. D-cycloserine

    C. Glutamate

    D. Glycine

40. **A meta-analysis of studies of mostly adult patients looking at pharmacological treatment of generalized anxiety disorder found what effect size for benzodiazepines?**

    A. 0.18

    B. 0.38

    C. 1.88

    D. There was no effect.

41. **A therapeutic alliance in adult psychotherapy is usually established after how many sessions?**

    A. 1 or 2

    B. 3 to 5

    C. 5 to 7

    D. 7 to 10

42. **What is a discontinuation trial?**

    A. After double-blind treatment, subjects are randomly and blindly assigned to active treatment or placebo.

    B. After double-blind treatment, subjects are randomly and openly assigned to active treatment or placebo.

    C. After open-label treatment, subjects are randomly and blindly assigned to active treatment or placebo.

    D. After double-blind treatment, subjects are discontinued.

43. Antidepressants to treat major depressive disorder in children and adolescents with comorbid epilepsy:

    A. Have no effect on mood

    B. Worsen the frequency of seizures

    C. Decrease the frequency of seizures

    D. Improve depressive symptoms

44. An obsessive and restless agitation can be found in severely emaciated patients, such as those with anorexia. This is likely related to:

    A. Bone density loss

    B. Bradycardia

    C. Electrolyte imbalance

    D. Leptin deficiency

45. What fraction of pregnancies in the United States are unplanned?

    A. A tenth

    B. An eighth

    C. A quarter

    D. Half

46. Studies have consistently shown that reports from behavior checklists and questionnaires used to clarify diagnosis or determine the severity of psychiatric illness are most valid from which source?

    A. Teachers

    B. Parents

    C. The patient

    D. None of the above

47. When switching from an antipsychotic that has strongly antihistaminic properties to one that has minimal histamine blocking, all of the following may occur EXCEPT:

    A. Hypersomnolence

    B. Anxiety

    C. Agitation

    D. EPS

    E. Restlessness

48. At what age is the mean peak volume of the cerebral cortical gray matter attained?

    A. 18 years

    B. 12 years

    C. 8 years

    D. 6 years

    E. 4 years

49. All the following have been reported as side effects of selective serotonin reuptake inhibitor (SSRI) treatment. Which is frequently seen in children?

    A. Extrapyramidal symptoms

    B. Amotivational syndrome

    C. Behavioral activation

    D. Impaired clotting

50. Which of the following is a side effect of atomoxetine?

    A. Decrease in blood pressure

    B. Increase in suicidal thinking

    C. Decrease in heart rate

    D. Electrocardiogram changes

51. Which of the following groups would be considered "vulnerable" from a research perspective?

    A. Elderly woman

    B. Adult woman

    C. Prisoner

    D. 18-year-old man

52. In what decade were tricyclic antidepressants discovered to be effective in the treatment of depression?

    A. 1920s

    B. 1940s

    C. 1950s

    D. 1970s

53. Which of the following statements about disclosure of financial or other relationships with drug companies is accurate?

    A. Disclosure reduces bias.

    B. Non-disclosure undermines the trust of patients or colleagues.

    C. Disclosure satisfies conflict-of-interest requirements.

    D. Non-disclosure increases bias.

54. Which category of antidepressant medications does venlafaxine occupy based on its mechanism of action?

    A. Selective serotonin/norepinephrine reuptake inhibitors (SNRI)

    B. Selective serotonin reuptake inhibitors (SSRI)

    C. Tricyclic antidepressant (TCA)

    D. Exact mechanism of action is unknown.

55. Which of the following side effects may occur with the use of benzodiazepines?

    A. Anterograde amnesia

    B. Sialorrhea

    C. Disinhibition

    D. Autonomic instability

    E. A and C

56. In what decade did mirtazapine emerge as a treatment for depression?

    A. 1930s

    B. 1950s

    C. 1970s

    D. 1990s

57. Fluvoxamine has FDA approval for what disorder in children?

    A. Obsessive-compulsive disorder (OCD)

    B. Major depressive disorder (MDD)

    C. Generalized anxiety disorder (GAD)

    D. Posttraumatic stress disorder (PTSD)

58. The lack of FDA approval for the use of a medication for a disorder suggests:

    A. The medication is contraindicated for treatment of the disorder.

    B. The medication is somewhat contraindicated for treatment of the disorder.

    C. The medication is absolutely contraindicated for treatment of the disorder.

    D. None of the above

59. Which of the following has been shown to be no better than placebo for control of tics?

    A. Haloperidol

    B. Risperidone

    C. Ziprasidone

    D. Clozapine

60. What percentage of children and adolescents diagnosed with attention-deficit/hyperactivity disorder (ADHD) are prescribed stimulants?

    A. 30%

    B. 50%

    C. 70%

    D. 90%

61. In a follow-up of 45 patients, childhood factors associated with the persistence of obsessive-compulsive disorder (OCD) symptoms into adulthood included:

    A. Male gender

    B. Absence of tics

    C. Absence of hoarding symptoms

    D. Good sleep hygiene

    E. Absence of major depression

62. Which of the following reflects the physician's cardinal rule of *primum non nocere*, first do no harm?

    A. Autonomy

    B. Justice

    C. Nonmaleficence

    D. Beneficence

63. Alpha-2 agonist inhibition of kindling in the amygdalohippocampal area might suggest a possible role for alpha agonists in the treatment of what disorder in particular?

    A. Schizophrenia

    B. Somatization disorder

    C. Pain disorder

    D. Posttraumatic stress disorder

64. Although it is not uniformly accepted, most investigators believe the treatment effect of serotonergic agents in obsessive-compulsive disorder (OCD) is mediated by:

    A. Up-regulation of alpha-2 autoreceptors

    B. Down-regulation of post-synaptic 5-HT$_{2A}$ receptors

    C. Up-regulation of post-synaptic 5-HT$_3$ receptors

    D. Down-regulation of the presynaptic 5-HT$_{1D}$ autoreceptor

65. What evidence supports the consideration that lamotrigine may possess antidepressant properties?

    A. It is a first-line treatment for major depressive disorder.

    B. It is a potent monoamine oxidase inhibitor.

    C. It inhibits serotonin reuptake.

    D. It has a synergistic effect with SSRIs.

    E. None of the above

66. What happens when a benzodiazepine binds the benzodiazepine receptor?

    A. The capacity of GABA to open chloride channels decreases.

    B. The capacity of GABA to open chloride channels increases.

    C. The capacity of GABA to open calcium channels decreases.

    D. The capacity of GABA to open calcium channels increases.

67. Which of the following medications may cause prolonged seizures if used concomitantly with electroconvulsive therapy (ECT)?

    A. Trazodone

    B. Lithium

    C. Fluoxetine

    D. A and C

68. Angold and colleagues surveyed 1422 children and adolescents in North Carolina and found which of the following about attention-deficit/hyperactivity disorder (ADHD)?

    A. The majority of children who were prescribed stimulants did not meet their research criteria for ADHD.

    B. A large minority of children who were diagnosed with ADHD did not receive stimulants.

    C. Being young predicted stimulant use.

    D. Being male predicted stimulant use.

    E. All of the above

69. Withdrawal dyskinesias occur in which situation?

    A. When an SSRI is rapidly reduced or eliminated

    B. When an antipsychotic is rapidly reduced or eliminated

    C. When a benzodiazepine is rapidly reduced or eliminated

    D. None of the above

70. Should a neuropsychological assessment be performed in children as a component of electroconvulsive therapy (ECT)?

    A. Yes, prior to treatment and immediately after the treatment

    B. Yes, prior to treatment and 6 months after the treatment

    C. Yes, 2 months after treatment

    D. No, neuropsychological assessments are not recommended

71. Which of the following is the most prevalent neurotransmitter system in the human brain?

    A. Cholinergic

    B. Glutamatergic

    C. Dopaminergic

    D. Serotonergic

72. Treatment of which of the following has been shown to improve outcome in depressed youth?

    A. Falling academic performance

    B. Decreasing social participation

    C. Acute stress symptoms

    D. Parental depression

73. What has been observed in a small number of children with a family history of bipolar disorder who are started on guanfacine?

    A. Hypersomnolence

    B. Early-morning awakening

    C. Galactorrhea

    D. Hypomanic-like agitation

74. Which of the following medications is FDA-labeled for "severe explosive behaviors" in pediatric patients but is not generally used because of its side-effect profile?

    A. Thioridazine

    B. Olanzapine

    C. Aripiprazole

    D. Quetiapine

75. Among all patients with a substance-use disorder, which age group has the highest rates of co-occurring psychiatric disorders?

    A. 15 to 24 years of age

    B. 34 to 45 years of age

    C. 54 to 65 years of age

    D. 74 to 85 years of age

76. Which of the following antipsychotics has demonstrated a reduction in prolactin level upon administration?

    A. Risperidone

    B. Olanzapine

    C. Aripiprazole

    D. Ziprasidone

77. There is a dearth of scales for clinical trials in child and adolescent psychiatry in which one of the following areas?

    A. Anxiety

    B. Depression

    C. Functioning

    D. Attention-deficit/hyperactivity disorder

78. The Preschool ADHD Treatment Study (PATS) not only indicated a clinically and statistically significant difference between methylphenidate treatment and placebo in preschoolers with ADHD, but also indicated an improvement in which functional measures?

    A. Social competence

    B. Social skills

    C. Parenting stress

    D. All of the above

    E. None of the above

79. All the following are common structural brain abnormalities seen consistently in schizophrenia EXCEPT:

    A. Enlargement of the lateral and third ventricles

    B. Increased asymmetry of the basal ganglia

    C. Reduced total brain volume

    D. Reduced volume of the cortical gray matter

80. Common adverse effects of valproate include all the following EXCEPT:

    A. Weight gain

    B. Transient hair loss

    C. Renal dysfunction

    D. Thrombocytopenia

    E. Vomiting

81. Venlafaxine is FDA-approved for all of the following indications EXCEPT:

    A. Generalized anxiety disorder

    B. Panic disorder

    C. Social phobia

    D. Obsessive-compulsive disorder

82. Generally, how many SSRI trials should precede a clomipramine trial in the partially responsive child with obsessive-compulsive disorder (OCD)?

    A. 1

    B. 2

    C. 3

    D. B and C

83. What is the estimated lifetime incidence of physical and sexual abuse for child and adolescent psychiatric outpatients?

    A. 5%

    B. 15%

    C. 30%

    D. 45%

84. Neurosurgery in humans and other species has demonstrated that amygdalectomy and temporal lobectomy results in decreased:

    A. Memory

    B. Libidinal drive

    C. Aggression

    D. Impulse control

85. A starting dose of valproate at 15 mg per kilogram daily in children and adolescents will produce serum valproate levels in what range?

    A. 20 to 30 mg/mL

    B. 30 to 50 mg/mL

    C. 50 to 60 mg/mL

    D. 60 to 70 mg/mL

    E. 70 to 80 mg/mL

86. In one study, the factors associated with elevated thyroid-stimulating hormone (TSH) levels in children and adolescents treated with lithium included:

    A. Higher baseline TSH level

    B. Elevated glomerular filtration rate

    C. Higher lithium level

    D. Tremor

    E. A and C

87. Direct-to-consumer advertising is legal in which number of countries?

    A. 2

    B. 25

    C. 50

    D. 100

88. The tertiary amines, compared with the secondary amines, of tricyclic antidepressants are:

    A. More serotonergic

    B. More dopaminergic

    C. More noradrenergic

    D. More GABA-ergic

89. In obsessive-compulsive disorder, which group has the least insight?

    A. Children

    B. Adolescents

    C. Middle-aged adults

    D. Older adults

90. The binding of atypical antipsychotics to $5HT_{2A}$ receptors seems to be associated with which of the following?

    A. Less prolactin elevation

    B. Increased extrapyramidal symptoms

    C. Less growth hormone secretion

    D. Increased appetite

91. A randomized controlled trial of antihistamines for aggression in boys demonstrated which of the following?

    A. There is no difference between intramuscular and oral route.

    B. There is no difference between placebo and active agent.

    C. Physical aggression declined significantly.

    D. All of the above

92. At this time only three families of CYP enzymes have been shown to be involved in human metabolism of exogenous agents. These are:

    A. CYP1, CYP2, and CYP3

    B. CYP2, CYP4, and CYP5

    C. CYP2, CYP4, and CYP6

    D. CYP2, CYP4, and CYP8

93. What types of comparison groups can be used in randomized therapy trials?
    A. No treatment
    B. Placebo
    C. Dose-response
    D. Active control
    E. All of the above

94. Which of the following medications is useful for decreasing bladder contractility while increasing bladder outlet resistance in the treatment of pediatric enuresis?
    A. Scopolamine
    B. Imipramine
    C. Atropine
    D. DDAVP

95. All the following are reported side effects of pregabalin EXCEPT:
    A. Somnolence
    B. Weight loss
    C. Dizziness
    D. Headache
    E. Dry mouth

96. Which term describes functionally relevant modifications to the genome not involving a change in the DNA nucleotide sequence?
    A. Transcription
    B. Epigenetics
    C. Translation
    D. Triplet repeats

97. Which is the most efficacious intervention for children diagnosed with posttraumatic stress disorder (PTSD)?
    A. Eye movement desensitization and reprocessing (EMDR)
    B. Trauma-focused CBT
    C. Play therapy
    D. Family therapy

98. Which area of the brain has been implicated in the recognition of others' emotional states through the analysis of facial expressions?
    A. Lateral fusiform gyrus
    B. Nucleus accumbens
    C. Amygdala
    D. Globus pallidus pars interna

99. Which of the following agents has an extended-release formulation approved by the FDA for attention-deficit/hyperactivity disorder (ADHD)?
    A. Desipramine
    B. Atomoxetine
    C. Modafinil
    D. Guanfacine

100. For which of the following disorders is it difficult to develop indicated drugs because of the heterogeneity of the presentation?
    A. Major depressive disorder
    B. Schizophrenia
    C. Bipolar disorder
    D. Conduct disorder

101. Which of the following has been suggested by some for anxiety disorders?
    A. Peanuts
    B. Valerian
    C. Corn husk extract
    D. Secretin

102. Which of the following is a benzodiazepine hypnotic?
    A. Clorazepate
    B. Zolpidem
    C. Zaleplon
    D. Eszoplicone

103. Which type of bipolar disorder requires the presence of a manic or mixed episode?
    A. Bipolar I disorder
    B. Bipolar II disorder
    C. Cyclothymic disorder
    D. Bipolar disorder NOS

104. The following are side effects of stimulants. Which two are the most commonly reported?

A. Sleep disturbances and appetite suppression

B. Headaches and sleep disturbances

C. Abdominal discomfort and sleep disturbances

D. Mood disturbances and headaches

105. Most orally ingested drugs are absorbed at what anatomic location?

A. Stomach

B. Small intestine

C. Proximal large intestine

D. Distal large intestine

106. Increased activity from drug-associated cues in which area of the brain has been correlated with craving caused by drug paraphernalia or memories of drug use?

A. Hippocampus

B. Orbitofrontal cortex

C. Nucleus accumbens

D. Limbic system

107. Which of these is NOT a diagnostic subtype of ADHD?

A. Hyperactive-impulsive

B. Hyperactive

C. Inattentive

D. Combined

108. Presynaptic dopaminergic receptors are typically what type?

A. D_2

B. D_3

C. D_4

D. D_5

109. What is the prevalence of nocturnal enuresis for children 5 years of age?

A. 2%

B. 5%

C. 15%

D. 25%

110. What is the key component in determining the duration of action of each benzodiazepine?

A. Elimination half-life

B. Potency

C. Oxidation

D. Distribution half-life

111. All the following are common neuropsychological deficits in children with maladaptive aggression EXCEPT:

A. Disinhibition

B. Inability to learn from mistakes

C. Inability to anticipate consequences

D. Sensitivity to social cues

E. Impulsivity

112. In several countries the weight threshold criterion for anorexia nervosa in children and adolescents is what BMI percentile?

A. 1%

B. 5%

C. 10%

D. 15%

113. Which of the following describes the normal cardiovascular response during electroconvulsive therapy (ECT)?

A. Initial sympathetic outflow followed by parasympathetic outflow

B. Initial parasympathetic outflow followed by sympathetic outflow

C. Sympathetic outflow only

D. Parasympathetic outflow only

114. Which of the following has shown promise in the treatment of attention-deficit/hyperactivity disorder (ADHD)?

A. Nicotine

B. Glucocorticoids

C. Growth hormone

D. Levothyroxine

115. Since the 1990s tobacco use among children and adolescence has:

    A. Increased slightly

    B. Increased dramatically

    C. Remained the same

    D. Decreased

116. Which factor in children and adolescents with intellectual disability is associated with self-injurious behaviors?

    A. Age

    B. Severity of intellectual disability

    C. Deficits in communication abilities

    D. All of the above

117. In relation to citalopram, escitalopram is the:

    A. (R)-enantiomer

    B. Methylated estradiol group

    C. Pro-drug

    D. (S)-enantiomer

118. Which is the most commonly prescribed antidepressant in Germany?

    A. St. John's wort

    B. Fluvoxamine

    C. Venlafaxine

    D. Paroxetine

119. The Course and Outcome of Bipolar Illness in Youth (COBY) study found that approximately what percentage of youth with bipolar I disorder had a prior history of major depressive episode?

    A. 5%

    B. 12%

    C. 25%

    D. 50%

120. What is the estimated prevalence of the adverse effect of priapism in males treated with trazodone?

    A. 1 in 2000

    B. 1 in 4000

    C. 1 in 6000

    D. 1 in 8000

121. Most members of which of the following drug classes are $5\text{-}HT_2$ receptor antagonists?

    A. SSRIs

    B. Tricyclic antidepressants

    C. Atypical antipsychotics

    D. Benzodiazepines

122. All the following have been used synonymously with "conflict of interest" EXCEPT:

    A. Competing interest

    B. Dual commitment

    C. Competing loyalties

    D. Synergy

123. In conducting an assessment of a child, a psychiatrist learns that an uncle had the same disorder suspected in the child who committed suicide. What are some considerations the psychiatrist might have in working with the family?

    A. The family will be eager to prevent a similar outcome.

    B. The family may have trouble accepting the diagnosis.

    C. The family may have trouble accepting treatment.

    D. All of the above

124. If a medication change in a pregnant woman with a severe psychotic disorder is necessary, treatment with which medication is recommended?

    A. Clozapine

    B. Olanzapine

    C. Haloperidol

    D. Quetiapine

125. Which of the following is the type of question that explanatory clinical trials seek to answer?

    A. Does this intervention work under usual conditions?

    B. Does this intervention work under ideal conditions?

    C. Both statements

    D. None of the above

126. All of the following are thought to potentially play a role in tics EXCEPT:

    A. Androgens

    B. Psychological stress

    C. Body temperature regulation

    D. Myopia

    E. Group A beta-hemolytic streptococcus

127. Drugs have to exhibit a sufficient degree of what quality in order to be orally absorbed and distributed to receptors in the central nervous system?

    A. Hydrophilicity

    B. Lipophilicity

    C. Both

    D. None

128. Which of the following agents reversibly inhibits gastric and pancreatic lipase?

    A. Sibutramine

    B. Metoclopramide

    C. Orlistat

    D. Omeprazole

129. It is suggested that the clinician should obtain an EKG for a patient starting an antipsychotic when which of the following is present?

    A. At baseline for all patients

    B. When a patient is on other QTc-prolonging medications

    C. Family history of sudden cardiac death in first-degree relatives aged <65 for males and <70 for females

    D. Family history of irregular heartbeat

130. Which of the following physicochemical properties of a drug would likely result in favorable absorption?

    A. Non-polar, highly lipid-soluble, and small molecular size

    B. Non-polar, non-lipid-soluble, and medium molecular size

    C. Highly polar, non-lipid-soluble, and large molecular size

    D. None of the above

131. Patients on lamotrigine treatment also taking oral contraceptives require:

    A. Higher doses of lamotrigine

    B. Equivalent doses of lamotrigine

    C. Lower doses of lamotrigine

    D. Prompt discontinuation of lamotrigine

132. What is the level of evidence for buspirone use in children and adolescents?

    A. Two double-blind, randomized controlled trials showing positive effect for anxiety

    B. Two double-blind, randomized controlled trials showing positive effect for depression

    C. Two double-blind, randomized controlled trials showing positive effect for adjunctive use in anxiety

    D. There are no controlled studies in this age group.

133. Which two agents are least likely to lead to QTc prolongation or torsades de pointes?

    A. Ziprasidone and thioridazine

    B. Olanzapine and aripiprazole

    C. Olanzapine and risperidone

    D. Risperidone and quetiapine

134. Open-label trials of riluzole indicate a reduction of symptoms in unipolar and bipolar depression in adults by addressing which neurochemical target?

    A. Abnormal serotonergic concentrations

    B. Abnormal adrenergic concentrations

    C. Abnormal cholinergic concentrations

    D. Abnormal glutamatergic concentrations

135. Near-term *in utero* exposure to antipsychotic agents has been linked to which of the following symptoms in neonates?

    A. Neural tube defects

    B. Extrapyramidal symptoms

    C. Tardive dyskinesia

    D. Physiological withdrawal

136. Post-marketing studies to delineate additional information about a drug's risks, benefits and optimal use are called:

    A. Phase 0 trials

    B. Phase I trials

    C. Phase II trials

    D. Phase III trials

    E. Phase IV trials

137. At what age is the functioning of the prefrontal cortex (PFC) first evident?

    A. Birth

    B. 4 months

    C. 6 months

    D. 1 year

138. What percentage of children in foster care receive three or more different drug classes during a given year (not necessarily simultaneously)?

    A. <10%

    B. 20%

    C. 30%

    D. >40%

139. Which National Institutes of Health study examined the role of stimulant medications in the treatment of preschoolers?

    A. The Psychotropic 0 to 18 Study (P018 Study)

    B. The Multimodal Treatment Study for ADHD (MTA)

    C. The School-age Study for ADHD (SASA)

    D. The Preschool ADHD Treatment Study (PATS)

140. Most children display physically aggressive behaviors during infancy and subsequently learn alternative means of expression and interaction. At what period do children generally learn to regulate aggressive behaviors?

    A. Before entering toddlerhood

    B. Before entering preschool

    C. Before entering primary school

    D. Before entering secondary school

141. A 16-year-old girl develops signs of lithium toxicity. Which of the following is NOT a symptom of lithium toxicity?

    A. Fine tremor

    B. Nausea

    C. Slurred speech

    D. Vomiting

    E. Dyscoordination

142. The FDA subscribes to the standard provided by the International Conference on Harmonization (ICH) E-10 document to determine when a particular trial design is ethical. What is the criterion regarding placebo use?

    A. Placebo is indicated for controlled clinical trials when there are mechanisms in place for severely ill patients to receive treatment after the study.

    B. Given the response to placebo in pediatric psychopharmacology trials, another option should be used for the control arm.

    C. A placebo-controlled trial is unacceptable only if standard drugs exist that are effective in reducing either mortality or irreversible morbidity.

    D. Those receiving placebo should not be blinded to the treatment.

143. Memantine is a non-competitive antagonist of which of the following receptors?

    A. GABA

    B. NMDA

    C. NE

    D. DA

    E. 5-HT

144. The desmopressin acetate nasal spray used for pediatric nocturnal enuresis carries an FDA black box warning for its association with which adverse effect?

    A. Seizures

    B. Headaches

    C. Hypertension

    D. Hyponatremia

145. To assess for hyperglycemia, emerging diabetes, and dyslipidemia, all should be monitored during neuroleptic treatment EXCEPT:

    A. Glucose

    B. Total cholesterol

    C. Triglycerides

    D. Insulin

146. What is the approximate prevalence of bipolar disorder in adolescence?

    A. 0.2%

    B. 0.4%

    C. 1%

    D. 2%

147. Caloric replacement in severely malnourished anorexic patients must proceed slowly to avoid:

    A. Hypophosphatemia

    B. Increased intracellular fluid

    C. Decreased insulin

    D. Decreased oxygen consumption

148. Weight gain in children on antipsychotics appears greater than that found in adults on antipsychotics. What might be an explanation?

    A. Doses in children are much higher than in adults.

    B. Children have less healthy diets.

    C. Children have less prior antipsychotic use and thus less prior weight gain.

    D. Children are less adherent to their medication regimen than adults.

149. Melatonin for insomnia is generally regarded as safe; however, which of the following are potential adverse effects of the medication?

    A. Possible triggering of precocious puberty upon discontinuation

    B. Suppression of the hypothalamic-gonadal axis

    C. Increased reactivity of the immune system in children on immunosuppressants

    D. All of the above

150. Which of the following explains the advances in clinical research in pediatric pharmacotherapy?

    A. The doubling of research funding at the National Institutes of Health in the 1990s

    B. The Food and Drug Administration Modernization ACT (FDAMA) of 1997, which provided 6 months of additional market exclusivity for companies that conducted pediatric clinical trials

    C. The Pediatric Research Equity ACT (PREA), which required pharmaceutical companies to conduct pediatric studies of medications likely to be used by children and adolescents

    D. All of the above

151. What system does the FDA rely on to signal problems or potential problems with medications once they have come to market?

    A. Center for Drug Evaluation and Research

    B. Centers of Disease Control

    C. Emergency room reporting

    D. MedWatch

152. The addition of ketoconazole to a regimen that includes alprazolam is likely to lead to:

    A. Immediate toxicity

    B. Delayed toxicity

    C. No change in alprazolam levels

    D. Decrease in alprazolam levels

153. Findings from longitudinal studies indicate a relationship between the occurrence of separation anxiety disorder and what disorder subsequently?

    A. Major depression

    B. Bipolar disorder

    C. Panic attacks

    D. Dysthymia

154. Genetic polymorphisms play a role in each of these CYPs EXCEPT:

    A. CYP3A4

    B. CYP2D6

    C. CYP2C19

    D. CYP2C9

155. First-order elimination kinetics implies what kind of relationship between changes in dosage and plasma concentration?

    A. Inverse

    B. Parabolic

    C. Linear

    D. None of the above

156. Which of the following is a 5-HT$_{1a}$ agonist that may have a role in reducing anxiety, flashbacks, and insomnia in posttraumatic stress disorder (PTSD)?

    A. Sertraline

    B. Fluoxetine

    C. Buspirone

    D. Mirtazapine

157. A prospective observational cohort study found that preterm birth rates exceeded 20% for mothers who:

    A. Remained on an SSRI throughout pregnancy

    B. Suffered from untreated depression throughout pregnancy

    C. Both of the above

    D. None of the above

158. Which of the following was developed to screen for higher mental functions in psychiatric patients, and has been modified for use in children?

    A. Delirium Rating Scale

    B. Wechsler Adult Intelligence Scale

    C. Confusion Assessment Method

    D. Folstein Mini Mental State Exam

159. Due to FDA demands, the manufacturers of paroxetine added a warning regarding what potential teratogenic effects?

    A. Ebstein's anomaly

    B. Ventricular and atrial septal defects

    C. Neural tube defects

    D. Micrognathia

160. You are treating a 10-year-old with a selective serotonin reuptake inhibitor for her generalized anxiety and there has been no response with an adequate trial. Which of the following might be your next step?

    A. Switch to another SSRI.

    B. Cease medication treatment.

    C. Augment with levothyroxine.

    D. Switch to an SNRI.

161. The half-life of carbamazepine in children compared with adults is:

    A. Longer

    B. Similar

    C. Shorter

    D. Variable

162. Children and adolescents with major depressive disorder (MDD), subsequent to an acute positive response to antidepressant treatment, should continue treatment for at least what duration of time?

    A. 2 months

    B. 4 months

    C. 6 months

    D. 18 months

163. The likelihood of rapid-cycling bipolar disorder in children compared with adults is:

    A. Equivalent

    B. Increased

    C. Decreased

    D. Not present in children

164. In a randomized, controlled trial youths with major depressive disorder, conduct disorder, and substance-use disorder were randomized to cognitive behavioral therapy (CBT) and fluoxetine or placebo. Which statement accurately reflects the findings?

    A. Substance-use disorders improved most in the placebo group.

    B. Mood symptoms improved more in the fluoxetine group, but substance use was equal in both groups.

    C. Substance use improved in the fluoxetine group despite no improvement in mood.

    D. CBT was ineffective in both groups.

165. One of the largest published drug studies in autistic disorder reported what effect in the treatment of repetitive behaviors by citalopram in children and adolescents?

    A. Citalopram was no better than placebo in reducing repetitive behaviors.

    B. Citalopram was significantly better than placebo in reducing repetitive behaviors.

    C. The placebo was significantly better than citalopram in reducing repetitive behaviors.

    D. A dose-response relationship determines the effect of citalopram on repetitive behaviors.

166. What is the main reason clonidine should be tapered when it is discontinued?

    A. Rebound hypotension

    B. Rebound bradycardia

    C. Rebound diaphoresis

    D. Rebound hypertension

167. According to National Ambulatory Medical Care Survey data, the annual rate for psychotropic use in children was 1.4 per 100 persons in 1987. This number had increased to _____ per 100 persons by 1996.

    A. 1.7

    B. 3.9

    C. 10.5

    D. 22.3

168. Which term describes the clinical or research measure that generates a descriptive conclusion that is easily understood and practical?

    A. Face validity

    B. Continuous measure

    C. Categorical measure

    D. Dimensional measure

169. A patient who has failed to respond to two or three trials of antipsychotics is more likely to respond to which medication?

    A. Paliperidone

    B. Clozapine

    C. Quetiapine

    D. Olanzapine

170. St. John's wort has been used to treat all of the following disorders EXCEPT:

    A. Depression

    B. Tics

    C. ADHD

    D. Somatoform disorders

    E. Schizophrenia

171. Nicotinic receptors bind which of the following compounds?

    A. Acetylcholine

    B. Muscarine

    C. Pilocarpine

    D. Bethanechol

172. Aside from psychosocial interventions, what is the first line of approach for medication use in Tourette's disorder?

    A. Start medications as soon as possible when in the midst of a severely disruptive episode.

    B. Defer use of medications to see if the tics wane.

    C. Prescribe medications as needed (PRN).

    D. Prescribe an alpha agonist.

173. Which of the following statements is accurate?

    A. Informed consent is obtained before initiating a medication and is considered complete once the parents agree to the proposed treatment.

    B. The parents live with the behavior, so the risks of no treatment are not discussed usually as part of the consent process.

    C. Although guardians consent to treatment, having an adolescent assent to treatment helps ensure adherence and success.

    D. It is best to avoid discussions about the likely length of treatment, since the outcome is often unpredictable.

174. Anxiety disorders are more often comorbid than not. Which answer option characterizes the developmental progression of anxiety disorders?

    A. Obsessive-compulsive disorder, generalized anxiety disorder, social phobia, separation anxiety disorder

    B. Obsessive-compulsive disorder, separation anxiety disorder, social phobia, generalized anxiety disorder

    C. Separation anxiety disorder, generalized anxiety disorder, social phobia, obsessive-compulsive disorder

    D. Generalized anxiety disorder, obsessive-compulsive disorder, social phobia, separation anxiety disorder

175. An electroconvulsive therapy (ECT) treatment study on 72 adolescents indicated marked improvement or resolution of symptoms in half the adolescents who completed a course of ECT. Adolescent patients diagnosed with which psychiatric illness derived the most benefit?

    A. Oppositional defiant disorder

    B. Mood disorder

    C. Autism

    D. Personality disorder

176. Which of the following medications has been most associated with priapism?

    A. Mirtazapine

    B. Paroxetine

    C. Trazodone

    D. Escitalopram

177. Approximately how many multiples of the plasma half-life is required to reach steady-state concentration in first-order kinetics?

    A. One

    B. 2 to 3

    C. 4 to 5

    D. 8 to 10

178. The STAR*D study (Sequenced Treatment Alternatives to Relieve Depression), which enrolled more than 2000 persons, found which of the following about the serotonin transporter gene?

    A. The *s* allele homozygotes had greater antidepressant response.

    B. The *l* allele homozygotes had greater antidepressant response.

    C. The *l* allele homozygotic males had a greater antidepressant response.

    D. The study did not find any serotonin transporter variants to be associated with any efficacy phenotype.

179. Which of the following medications is FDA-approved for smoking cessation in adults?

    A. Mirtazapine

    B. Bupropion

    C. Venlafaxine

    D. Duloxetine

180. What percentage of children with Tourette's disorder continue to experience at least a moderate level of impairment in global functioning by the age of 20 years?

    A. 90%

    B. 70%

    C. 45%

    D. 20%

181. Melatonin has been shown to be effective for which specific diagnostic population when added to sleep hygiene?

    A. Attention-deficit/hyperactivity disorder

    B. Major depressive disorder

    C. Posttraumatic stress disorder

    D. Polysubstance dependence

182. Alpha-1 receptor stimulation in the prefrontal cortex results in:

    A. Enhanced functioning in the prefrontal cortex

    B. Reduced functioning in the prefrontal cortex

    C. No change

    D. There are no alpha-2 receptors in the prefrontal cortex.

183. Pharmaceutical industry and academic center relationships:

    A. Are inherently unethical

    B. Do not pose a conflict of interest

    C. Have led to important drug developments

    D. Have decreased in number since the 1980s

184. Which of the following cardiac or EKG parameters is a contraindication to using clomipramine?

    A. PR interval >200 msec

    B. QRS interval >120 msec

    C. Blood pressure >140 systolic or >90 diastolic; or heart rate >130 at rest

    D. QTc >450 msec or >30% increase of QTc over baseline

    E. All of the above

185. The overall response rate to stimulants from all group studies for school-age children or adolescents with intellectual disability diagnosed with ADHD was:

    A. 15%

    B. 36%

    C. 54%

    D. 77%

186. In order to use methadone in youths under 18 years of age, the clinician must:

    A. Obtain consent from the adolescent; there is an exception to parental consent for methadone treatment.

    B. Document two trials of methadone-free rehabilitation.

    C. Prescribe as soon as clinically indicated, just as in adults.

    D. Double the dose to accommodate increased metabolism.

187. Combining dextromethorphan (a potential ingredient of over-the-counter cough syrup) with which of the following medications may result in symptoms of serotonin syndrome?

    A. Fluoxetine

    B. Isocarboxazid

    C. Bupropion

    D. A and C

188. What has been identified as the cause of the majority of cases of Rett's disorder?

    A. Aspirin

    B. A mutation in the MeCP2 gene

    C. Chromosome 15 translocation

    D. Genetic deletion from chromosome 7

    E. Expansion of a trinucleotide gene sequence on the X chromosome

189. Which of the following statements is FALSE?

    A. The addition of behavioral therapy to stimulant treatment improved the outcome of children with ADHD and anxiety.

    B. One small study that involved the addition of an SSRI to stimulant treatment for children with ADHD and anxiety showed that stimulant treatment alone equaled combined treatment.

    C. Atomoxetine may be useful in treating children with co-occurring ADHD and anxiety.

    D. The presence of anxiety decreases the responsiveness to stimulant treatment in ADHD.

190. All of these have been associated with anxiety disorder in childhood EXCEPT:

    A. Schizophrenia

    B. Educational underachievement

    C. Substance use

    D. Suicide

191. Which of the following tricyclic antidepressants (TCAs) has been shown to be efficacious in the treatment of obsessive-compulsive disorder?

    A. Imipramine

    B. Amitriptyline

    C. Amoxapine

    D. Clomipramine

192. Among the following psychosocial interventions, which is more effective for bulimia nervosa?

    A. Nutritional counseling

    B. Psychodynamic psychotherapy

    C. Interpersonal therapy (IPT)

    D. Supportive therapy

193. How often do youths with early-onset schizophrenia spectrum disorders (EOSS) spontaneously report positive symptoms compared to adults with schizophrenia?

    A. More likely to report

    B. Just as likely to report

    C. Less likely to report

    D. Youths do not experience positive symptoms of schizophrenia.

194. What term describes the common but erroneous belief held by many study subjects that their personal best interests will be served by research participation because the investigators are health-care professionals who in general must be committed to good patient care?

    A. Therapeutic conflict of interest

    B. Therapeutic determinism

    C. Therapeutic idealization

    D. Therapeutic misconception

195. All of these are side effects of selective serotonin reuptake inhibitors (SSRIs) EXCEPT:

    A. Anhidrosis

    B. Bleeding

    C. Vivid dreams

    D. Tremors

    E. Diarrhea

196. Chlorpromazine was first used clinically in which decade?

    A. 1900s

    B. 1920s

    C. 1950s

    D. 1970s

197. What is the half-life of clonidine in children?

    A. 1 to 2 hours

    B. 8 to 12 hours

    C. 18 to 24 hours

    D. Over 24 hours

198. In the treatment of anxiety for children, what dosing regimen, regardless of half-life, has been recommended for benzodiazepines?

    A. Single daily dose

    B. Twice-daily dose

    C. Multiple daily doses

    D. None of the above

199. The hypnotic effect of benzodiazepines is mediated by their action at which receptor?

    A. H1

    B. Alpha-1

    C. $GABA_A$

    D. D2

    E. Alpha-2

200. There are exceptions to parental consent in which a minor may consent to treatment. All the following are situations in which a minor, in some states, may consent EXCEPT:

    A. Substance use treatment

    B. Sexually transmitted disease treatment

    C. A talented and gifted adolescent

    D. Birth control

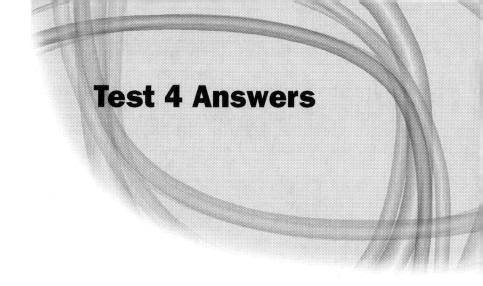

Test 4 Answers

1. Answer: D

Risperidone also appears to increase triglycerides. (Chap. 37)

2. Answer: B

Increased attention has been put on effect sizes rather than statistical significance as a way to focus on the clinical relevance of research results. (Chap. 50)

3. Answer: D

Approximately 20% of adolescents with ADHD will start smoking and 15% will develop other substance-use disorders. Stimulant treatment appears to reduce the risk. (Chap. 18)

4. Answer: D

Increased sensitivity of D2 dopamine receptors is suggested in Tourette's disorder. (Chap. 12)

5. Answer: B

Ondansetron (as well as granisetron) is an antagonist of the $5HT_3$ receptor and is a potent anti-emetic. (Chap. 2)

6. Answer: C

400 mg of EPA and 200 mg of DHA is the recommended dose for children. Fish oils need to be purchased from reputable companies that certify that the supplements are free of contaminants. (Chap. 25)

7. Answer: D

Trials of amitriptyline, desipramine, and nortriptyline all indicated improvement in symptoms for children with ADHD. (Chap. 21)

8. Answer: A and D

IPSRT is a manual-based therapy focusing on stabilizing social and sleep routines, the bidirectional relationship between moods and interpersonal events, and addressing interpersonal precipitants of dysregulation. (Chap. 33)

9. Answer: C

The consistent MRI findings are increased subcortical volume and decreased frontal cortex volume. (Chap. 11)

10. Answer: D

Significant hypoleptinemia occurs with depletion of fat stores and in acute anorexia nervosa usually triggers amenorrhea as the secretion of luteinizing and follicle-stimulating hormone depends on critical serum leptin thresholds. Studies show that hypoleptinemia induces hyperactivity. In patients with anorexia nervosa, hyperactivity levels are inversely correlated with serum leptin levels. (Chap. 16)

11. Answer: B

The rates of eating disorders are elevated in females, with an onset primarily in the second decade of life. (Chap. 16)

12. Answer: B

The Pediatric Research Equity Act and its predecessor, the Pediatric Rule, stipulated that a sponsor must have a pediatric study if the submission for a new drug application contained a new ingredient, indication, dosage form, dosing regimen, or route of administration. There is one exception to the PREA requirements: indications that have received orphan status (drug development for rare conditions) are exempt from PREA requirements. (Chap. 51)

13. Answer: B

An effect size of 0.5 is considered of medium magnitude. (Chap. 29)

14. Answer: A

Reliability describes the consistency of a screening or diagnostic instrument from one administration to another and from one rater to another. (Chap. 28)

15. Answer: D

Amphetamines have several mechanisms of action affecting the reuptake and release of catecholamines. (Chap. 31)

16. Answer: D

The duration of symptoms is 1 year compared to 2 years in adults. Two additional criterion symptoms need to be met to diagnose dysthymic disorder in children. (Chap. 32)

17. Answer: B

The rest of the MAOIs are non-selective irreversible inhibitors. (Chap. 21)

18. Answer: D

The presence of psychosis in patients with a prepubertal onset of bipolar disorder predicts a longer duration of mania or hypomania. (Chap. 33)

19. Answer: D

If whistle blowing occurs unethically or is resorted to with undue haste, reputations can be sullied by inaccurate or malicious accusations. (Chap. 53)

20. Answer: D

The maintenance phase of treatment for MDD, occurring after the 12-week acute phase and 6- to 12-month continuation phase, is intended to continue treatment for those with recurrent depression for 12 months or longer. (Chap. 32)

21. Answer: B

CYP enzymes oxidize drugs to more readily excretable forms in phase I metabolism. (Chap. 6)

22. Answer: E

Although pharmacological interventions are more rapid and potent, non-pharmacological treatments have been shown to have more long-lasting effects. Environmental measures include adjusting room temperature, and physiological measures include monitoring caffeine use. (Chap. 46)

23. Answer: D

It takes approximately 14 days for aripiprazole to reach steady-state plasma levels; it is important to take into account the pharmacokinetic and pharmacodynamic variability between different antipsychotic agents when assessing response. (Chap. 37)

24. Answer: D

High-dose lorazepam is indicated. If lorazepam is ineffective, ECT should be considered. (Chap. 43)

25. Answer: A

Cognitive deficits are lower with unilateral ECT and may also be lower when using ultra-brief-pulse ECT. (Chap. 26)

26. Answer: B

The clinical effect of immediate-release AMPH and MPH lasts about 4 hours. (Chap. 18)

27. Answer: B

Discontinuation syndrome may occur with mirtazapine, so a taper is recommended. (Chap. 21)

28. Answer: A

Up to 50% of youths who have a prescription will have two or more in the United States, especially youths diagnosed with bipolar disorder. The lowest prevalence is 6%, in Italy. (Chap. 54)

29. Answer: B

Whether the treatment is effective in reversing functional impairment is a reasonable question. The other questions would not be appropriate for a clinical trial. (Chap. 50)

30. Answer: C and D

Metabolism and excretion are primarily responsible for terminating the action of the pharmacologic agent upon the body. (Chap. 3)

31. Answer: A

After a drug company has done sufficient chemistry to have a drug substance suitable for human testing and has completed enough preclinical studies, it submits an application of an Investigational New Drug to the FDA. (Chap. 51)

32-B, 33-A, 34-C, 35-D. (Chap. 2)

36. Answer: D

Greater than 500 ms or an increase in the QTc over baseline of >60 msec is considered pathological. QTc dispersion (variance of QTc across at least six different leads) >100 msec might in fact be more relevant for the risk of arrhythmias, although this has not been thoroughly studied. (Chap. 23)

37. Answer: E

All of the listed medications can decrease REM stage sleep. (Chap. 46)

38. Answer: A

Tachypnea (with or without fever), tachycardia, panic, anxiety, and acute mental status changes can occur on abrupt discontinuation. Rebound hypertension is another consideration. (Chap. 19)

39. Answer: A

PCP also blocks the NMDA receptor inducing psychotic symptoms. D-cycloserine and glycine increase NMDA receptor function and have been reported to decrease psychotic and/or negative symptoms in schizophrenia. (Chap. 2)

40. Answer: B

One meta-analytic study in mostly adult patients found the effect size for benzodiazepines in GAD to be 0.38. (Chap. 24)

41. Answer: B

The relatively early establishment of a therapeutic alliance in adult psychotherapy may also have bearing on work with parents in child psychiatry. (Chap. 30)

42. Answer: C

A discontinuation study is a parallel group design in which patients are randomly and blindly assigned after open treatment. In this design relapse or recurrence of symptoms is the primary outcome variable. (Chap. 50)

43. Answer: D

Antidepressants in pediatric patients with comorbid seizures respond to antidepressants without an increase in seizure risk. (Chap. 43)

44. Answer: D

Patients with anorexia are often active to lose weight, but severely emaciated patients may be restless and obsessively agitated as a result of leptin deficiency. (Chap. 40)

45. Answer: D

More than half of pregnancies are unplanned, emphasizing the need for physicians to educate women regarding the potential obstetric and fetal risks associated with untreated mental illness as well as the risks of psychotropic medications. (Chap. 44)

46. Answer: B

The parent report has greater validity than youth or teacher report, even when the parent has a diagnosed mood disorder. (Chap. 33)

47. Answer: A

Insomnia may result from histamine rebound and not hypersomnolence. (Chap. 23)

48. Answer: B

The mean peak volume of cerebral cortical gray matter is reached at age 12 and then begins to decrease. (Chap. 1)

49. Answer: C

It may have a delayed onset that parallels the reduction in symptoms and may follow a honeymoon period of rapid improvement. (Chap. 35)

50. Answer: B

Warnings about suicidal thoughts and behaviors that apply to antidepressants also apply to atomoxetine. (Chap. 31)

51. Answer: C

Participants who have limited autonomy or are less than fully able to give proper informed consent on their own behalf are considered vulnerable. These include children, adults with impaired decision-making capacity, pregnant women and fetuses, and prisoners. Other vulnerable populations may include students, house staff, and employees of institutions conducting the research, illiterate subjects, and non-English-speaking subjects. (Chap. 52)

52. Answer: C

The effectiveness of tricyclic antidepressants for depression was discovered in the 1950s. (Chap. 21)

53. Answer: B

Disclosure per se does not reduce bias or influence, but non-disclosure undermines trust of patients or colleagues. (Chap. 53)

54. Answer: A

Venlafaxine is an SNRI. (Chap. 21)

55. Answer: E

Benzodiazepines can cause anterograde amnesia and disinhibited behaviors. (Chap. 46)

56. Answer: D

Mirtazapine emerged as a treatment for depression in the 1990s. (Chap. 21)

57. Answer: A

Fluvoxamine has FDA approval for OCD in children ages 8 to 17 and there are controlled data showing its efficacy in social phobia, separation anxiety, and GAD. (Chap. 20)

58. Answer: D

The lack of FDA approval for the use of a medication does not necessarily suggest a contraindication for its use. (Chap. 45)

59. Answer: D

Clozapine was not better than placebo in an early trial, suggesting that D2 antagonism is required for tic control. Risperidone, haloperidol, and ziprasidone, among others, have been shown to be effective for tics. (Chap. 36)

60. Answer: B

Approximately half of children diagnosed with ADHD receive a stimulant at some time. (Chap. 18)

61. Answer: B

In this study, the absence of tics was associated with a worse prognosis for treatment. Other risk factors for a poor prognosis were the presence of oppositional defiant disorder, prominent hoarding symptoms, female gender, later onset, and increased severity of OCD. (Chap. 11)

62. Answer: C

Nonmaleficence refers to doing no harm. (Chap. 52)

63. Answer: D

Alpha-agonist inhibition of kindling in the amygdalohippocampal area suggests a role in the treatment of post-traumatic stress disorder. (Chap. 19)

64. Answer: D

Down-regulation of the presynaptic 5-HT$_{1D}$ autoreceptor is thought to be the method by which SSRIs work in OCD. (Chap. 35)

65. Answer: C

Lamotrigine inhibits serotonin reuptake. (Chap. 22)

66. Answer: B

The capacity of GABA to open chloride channels increases when benzodiazepines bind to the receptor; this decreases cellular excitability, leading to an inhibitory effect. (Chap. 24)

67. Answer: D

Concomitant use of lithium with ECT may cause potentiation of the barbiturate and succinylcholine used in the procedure, or organic brain syndrome, but not prolonged seizures. (Chap. 26)

68. Answer: E

This question in part underscores the issue of "under" or "over" prescription in ADHD. Many of the children who did not meet criteria for ADHD received stimulants. However, only parent and child reports were used for diagnosis, and for children who had received stimulants but did not meet the criteria for diagnosis, high levels of ADHD symptoms were still found. In addition, teacher reports, which were not used in diagnosis, also indicated high levels of ADHD symptoms. (Chap. 49)

69. Answer: B

Withdrawal dyskinesias occur when an antipsychotic is rapidly reduced or eliminated. (Chap. 37)

70. Answer: B

When possible, neuropsychological assessments for children undergoing ECT should be performed prior to the

onset of treatment and 6 months after completion of ECT. (Chap. 26)

71. Answer: B

Both the glutamatergic and the GABA-ergic systems are the most prevalent and widely distributed neurotransmitters. (Chap. 2)

72. Answer: D

Treatment of parental depression improves treatment outcome in childhood depression. (Chap. 32)

73. Answer: D

This was observed in 5 of 95 children who received guanfacine in a psychopharmacology clinic. (Chap. 36)

74. Answer: A

Haloperidol, thioridazine, droperidone, and chlorpromazine have labeling for "severe explosive behaviors" in pediatric patients, although their clinical utility in actual practice is another matter. (Chap. 47)

75. Answer: A

Patients with substance-use disorders who are 15 to 24 years old have the highest rates of co-occurring psychiatric disorders. (Chap. 41)

76. Answer: C

Aripiprazole can lead to a decrease in prolactin level. Risperidone causes the greatest increase in prolactin level. (Chap. 37)

77. Answer: C

The dearth of scales that quantify level of functioning and that are sensitive to treatment effects is one of the major limitations of the current clinical trial methodology. (Chap. 50)

78. Answer: E

Only 21% of preschool children with ADHD in PATS reached remission at their optimal dose, and there was NO difference in functional measures compared with preschoolers on placebo. (Chap. 45)

79. Answer: B

Most structural abnormalities of the brain in schizophrenia have been found in first-episode, medication-naïve adults, implying they are not a consequence of damage from chronic disorder or treatment. (Chap. 13)

80. Answer: C

Common adverse effects of valproate include weight gain, transient hair loss, thrombocytopenia, vomiting, sedation, and tremor. (Chap. 22)

81. Answer: D

Venlafaxine is also FDA-approved for major depressive disorder. (Chap. 21)

82. Answer: D

According to experts, a child should have two or three trials of SSRIs prior to a clomipramine trial for partially responsive OCD. (Chap. 29)

83. Answer: C

Approximately one-third of child psychiatric outpatients are victims of abuse. (Chap. 8)

84. Answer: C

Temporal lobe removal was first reported to have a taming effect in animals in the 1890s. (Chap. 15)

85. Answer: C

Once this serum level of valproate is attained, which is considered subtherapeutic, the dose is often titrated upward, depending on tolerability and response. (Chap. 22)

86. Answer: E

A higher baseline TSH level and higher lithium levels may lead to elevated TSH while on lithium. Monitoring of thyroid function is recommended every 6 months or when clinically indicated in children and adolescents on lithium. (Chap. 22)

87. Answer: A

The United States and New Zealand permit direct-to-consumer advertising. No media (whether professional journals, television, radio or print media) can use prescription advertising in most Western European countries. (Chap. 54)

88. Answer: A

The tertiary amines are more serotonergic and the secondary amines are more noradrenergic. (Chap. 21)

89. Answer: A

Close to 20% of children have poor insight into their obsessions and compulsions. This compares to 6% in adolescents and adults. (Chap. 35)

90. Answer: A

Blockade of $5HT_{2A}$ receptors seems to be associated with less prolactin elevation and fewer extrapyramidal symptoms. (Chap. 23)

91. Answer: D

There was no difference in effect between placebo or active agent. Oral and IM routes were generally equivalent,

although the trend was for greater improvement with IM administration. (Chap. 47)

92. Answer: A

CYP3A metabolizes more than 40% to 50% of drugs, and it can do so in the small intestine or liver. In psychiatry, the most relevant CYP enzymes are CYP1A2, CYP2C9, CYP2C19, CYP2D6, and CYP3A4. (Chap. 4)

93. Answer: E

Pharmacotherapy trials can use several types of comparison groups, including no treatment, placebo, dose-response, and active control. (Chap. 50)

94. Answer: B

Imipramine has both central and peripheral anticholinergic effects. Atropine suppresses smooth muscle function but has considerable side effects. (Chap. 48)

95. Answer: B

There is a high likelihood of dose-dependent weight gain, and weight should be monitored. (Chap. 22)

96. Answer: B

Epigenetic modifications regulate gene activity through mechanisms such as DNA methylation and histone acetylation. (Chap. 8)

97. Answer: B

TF-CBT has been shown to be more effective than the other options. (Chap. 39)

98. Answer: C

The amygdala has a significant role in directing the visual system to seek out, fixate, attend to, and process affect-related stimuli found in facial expressions. (Chap. 14)

99. Answer: D

Guanfacine extended-release (Intuniv) is approved for the treatment of ADHD in children and adolescents. (Chap. 19)

100. Answer: D

Conduct disorder is unique in that it consists of a listing of behaviors that either violate the rights of others or in some other way violate societal norms. Thus, it is a disorder that is defined by the distress and dysfunction it causes to others, rather than to the individual with the diagnosis. In addition, the criteria can be met in a number of combinations, which can lead to a heterogeneous population. (Chap. 51)

101. Answer: B

There are studies of the anti-anxiety effect of valerian in adults and observational studies in children, but it is unclear whether these results can be generalized to anxiety disorders. As such, there is no evidence to recommend it at this stage. *(Chap. 25)*

102. Answer: A

Clorazepate is a benzodiazepine; zolpidem, zaleplon, and eszoplicone are non-benzodiazepine hypnotics. (Chap. 24)

103. Answer: A

Bipolar disorder I requires a manic or mixed episode. (Chap. 33)

104. Answer: A

Sleep disturbances and appetite suppression are the most commonly reported, with headaches and abdominal discomfort also common, however. (Chap. 31)

105. Answer: B

Most drugs are absorbed through the small intestine before entering the portal vein to the liver. (Chap. 4)

106. Answer: B

Cue-induced increased activity in the orbitofrontal cortex has been correlated with drug cravings. (Chap. 17)

107. Answer: B

The DSM does not recognize a hyperactive-only subtype. (Chap. 31)

108. Answer: A

Presynaptic D_2 receptors are autoreceptors that regulate dopamine synthesis and release as well as the firing rate of dopaminergic neurons. (Chap. 2)

109. Answer: C

The prevalence of nocturnal enuresis at the age of 5 is 15%. The rate of spontaneous remission of nocturnal enuresis is 15% per year thereafter. (Chap. 48)

110. Answer: D

Benzodiazepines are distributed until over 95% of the drug is outside the blood circulation, and the distribution half-life is thus most important in determining duration of action; however, elimination half-life is most studied. (Chap. 24)

111. Answer: D

Individuals with maladaptive aggression do not have high sensitivity to social cues, often making negative attributions. (Chap. 47)

112. Answer: C

BMI below 10% is the weight threshold for AN in several countries and corresponds roughly to the DSM-IV-TR weight criterion, 85% of expected body weight. A weight below 3% may warrant consideration of inpatient or day treatment. (Chap. 40)

113. Answer: B

The usual cardiovascular response to ECT consists of parasympathetic outflow (with bradycardia and asystole) followed by sympathetic outflow (with tachycardia, dysrhythmias, and hypertension). (Chap. 26)

114. Answer: A

Transdermal nicotine has been studied, as has a cholinergic nicotinic drug, ABT-148, which has structural similarities to nicotine. (Chap. 31)

115. Answer: D

Tobacco use has decreased among youths since the 1990s. (Chap. 41)

116. Answer: D

The risk of engaging in self-injurious behaviors appears higher during adolescence and young adulthood. (Chap. 42)

117. Answer: D

Escitalopram is the (S)-enantiomer of citalopram. (Chap. 20)

118. Answer: A

St. John's wort is the most commonly prescribed antidepressant in Germany. (Chap. 25)

119. Answer: D

The majority of youths with bipolar disorder present with depression as their index episode. Moreover, prepubertal children who present with major depressive disorder have an increased risk for subsequently developing bipolar disorder. (Chap. 33)

120. Answer: C

The estimated prevalence of priapism with trazodone is 1 in 6000 males. (Chap. 21)

121. Answer: C

Atypical antipsychotics are 5-HT_2 receptor antagonists, among other actions. (Chap. 2)

122. Answer: D

A number of terms are used synonymously with conflict of interest, but synergy is not one. (Chap. 53)

123. Answer: D

The family would not want their child to have a similar outcome, but they may have trouble accepting the diagnosis out of fear of the implications, and they may have trouble accepting the treatment for similar reasons or because they blamed the outcome on the treatment. (Chap. 27)

124. Answer: C

Haloperidol has not been associated with teratogenesis and possesses only a small risk for extrapyramidal symptoms in the newborn. (Chap. 44)

125. Answer: B

Randomized clinical trials have been broadly categorized as having either a pragmatic or explanatory approach. (Chap. 29)

126. Answer: D

Myopia has not been implicated in tic development. (Chap. 12)

127. Answer: B

Lipophilicity is necessary to a degree for a drug to be orally absorbed and distributed to receptors in the CNS. (Chap. 3)

128. Answer: C

Orlistat interferes with the catalyzing of triglycerides into absorbable free fatty acids. Orlistat has FDA approval for obesity in patients >12 years of age. (Chap. 40)

129. Answer: B

An EKG is obtained when other QTc-prolonging medications are prescribed or there is a risk factor for ventricular arrhythmias. Risk factors include family history of sudden cardiac death in first-degree relatives (males age <50, females <55), family history of prolonged QT syndrome, or a personal history of heart murmur, irregular heartbeat, tachycardia at rest, dizziness, or syncope on exertion. (Chap. 23)

130. Answer: A

A non-polar and lipid-soluble drug with a small molecular size is more readily absorbed than one with the opposite qualities. (Chap. 3)

131. Answer: A

Estrogen induces the metabolism of lamotrigine, so patients taking certain OCPs may require higher doses of lamotrigine. (Chap. 22)

132. Answer: D

The evidence for buspirone remains largely anecdotal for children and adolescents. In adults, there are controlled trials of buspirone showing a positive effect for anxiety. (Chap. 24)

133. Answer: B

Olanzapine and aripiprazole have not been found to lead to QTc prolongation or torsades de pointes in overdose. Thioridazine and ziprasidone have been found to lead to the most prolongation. (Chap. 43)

134. Answer: D

Riluzole may be effective in reducing symptoms of depression by targeting abnormal glutamatergic concentrations. (Chap. 9)

135. Answer: B

Signs of neonatal extrapyramidal symptoms (EPS) include hypertonicity, tremulousness, opisthotonus, torticollis, exaggerated deep tendon reflexes, and irritability. EPS are usually transient, lasting only days. (Chap. 44)

136. Answer: E

Phase IV trials usually involve comparisons between treatments that have already proven efficacious, or a company seeking approval for a new indication. (Chap. 50)

137. Answer: C

PFC functioning is first evident at 6 months of age. (Chap. 11)

138. Answer: D

It will vary by state and locale, but up to 40% of children in foster care will receive three or more different drug classes in a given year. (Chap. 49)

139. Answer: D

PATS examined 303 subjects aged 3 to 5.5 years. Options A and C (P018 and SASA) are fictitious. (Chap. 18)

140. Answer: C

Children generally learn to regulate aggression during the preschool years before entering primary school. (Chap. 15)

141. Answer: A

A fine tremor is a common adverse effect in children and adolescents and is not a sign of lithium toxicity. A coarse tremor would be a concern. (Chap. 22)

142. Answer: C

A placebo is unacceptable if there are other treatments available for a condition in which mortality or severe morbidity is a high risk. Because this is not the case in pediatric psychopharmacology, the FDA views placebo-controlled trials as acceptably safe and therefore ethical. (Chap. 51)

143. Answer: B

NMDA is a subclass of a glutamate receptor. (Chap. 38)

144. Answer: A

The black box warning is for the nasal spray's association with seizures and death, although all the listed options are potential adverse effects of desmopressin acetate. (Chap. 48)

145. Answer: D

HDL-cholesterol, LDL-cholesterol, blood glucose, and lipids should be measured at baseline and periodically thereafter. Insulin is not measured. (Chap. 23)

146. Answer: C

The prevalence of bipolar disorder in prepubertal children is 0.2% to 0.4%. (Chap. 9)

147. Answer: A

In refeeding syndrome, with the increased glucose load and insulin release resulting from eating, phosphate and other nutrients quickly enter the intracellular space, depleting the serum levels of phosphate. Phosphorus is required in the synthesis of many phosphorylated compounds, and its depletion can lead to serious problems in multiple organs. (Chap. 40)

148. Answer: C

Less prior antipsychotic use and therefore less prior weight gain may explain the apparent increased weight gain in children. This is suggested by a similar degree of large weight gain in antipsychotic-naïve adults. (Chap. 23)

149. Answer: D

Melatonin suppression of the hypothalamic-gonadal axis can potentially trigger precocious puberty upon discontinuation. (Chap. 46)

150. Answer: D

All of the answer options explain the growth in research in pediatric pharmacotherapy. (Chap. 27)

151. Answer: D

The FDA has a voluntary (spontaneous reporting) system that depends on clinicians and others (e.g., patients) to report adverse events to the FDA's MedWatch system. (Chap. 51)

152. Answer: B

There are two patterns of drug interactions, one with immediate effects and one with delayed effects, the latter occurring as the additional, inhibiting drug is co-administered regularly and reaches steady state. For drugs with high presystemic clearance (i.e., most of the drug is metabolized before reaching the systemic circulation), an inhibitor may lead to immediately increased levels. Alprazolam has low presystemic clearance, and therefore when an inhibitor is added little change in plasma concentration will occur after the first pass. (Chap. 4)

153. Answer: C

Family studies also indicate that childhood separation anxiety disorder relates to subsequent adult panic disorder. (Chap. 10)

154. Answer: A

The genetic variations lead to a lack of expression of CYP proteins, leading to poor CYP metabolic activity. Approximately 5% to 10% of all Caucasians are referred to as poor CYP2D6 metabolizers. One-fifth of Asians are genetically deficient in CYP2C19. (Chap. 4)

155. Answer: C

Linear kinetics in elimination means a constant fraction of drug is eliminated independent of the amount circulating in the bloodstream. (Chap. 3)

156. Answer: C

Buspirone has no controlled data in children but may be helpful in reducing anxiety, flashbacks, and insomnia. (Chap. 39)

157. Answer: C

This study provides additional evidence that untreated maternal depression can have adverse effects independent of antidepressant treatment. (Chap. 44)

158. Answer: D

The MMSE was developed as a screen for higher mental functions in psychiatric patients, although it is largely used as a dementia screen. It has been modified for use in the pediatric population. (Chap. 43)

159. Answer: B

Whether paroxetine actually does increase the risk of cardiac septal defects remains controversial. (Chap. 44)

160. Answer: A

The best evidence suggests switching to another SSRI. (Chap. 34)

161. Answer: C

The half-life of carbamazepine in children is between 8 and 14 hours, while in adults it is between 12 and 17 hours. (Chap. 22)

162. Answer: C

Children with MDD who responded to treatment should continue with it for at least 6 to 12 months. (Chap. 32)

163. Answer: B

Compared with adults, children are more likely to have mixed or rapid-cycling bipolar disorder. (Chap. 42)

164. Answer: B

In a trial by Riggs and associates, the fluoxetine group reported improved symptoms over the placebo group, but this did not have an impact on substance use; both groups, fluoxetine + CBT and placebo + CBT, had an average of 4 days of decreased use over 30 days. (Chap. 41)

165. Answer: A

The study, King et al. (2009), also found that citalopram was significantly more likely than placebo to be associated with adverse effects. (Chap. 38)

166. Answer: D

Clonidine should be tapered when it is discontinued to avoid rebound hypertension. (Chap. 19)

167. Answer: B

There has been an increase in the rate of prescriptions to children. In another survey the number of visits to ambulatory care that resulted in a prescription went from 1.10 million in 1985 to 3.73 million in 1993-94. (Chap. 49)

168. Answer: C

Categorical measures are usually dichotomous (e.g., responder or non-responder to exposure), but these measures can also have more than one category. (Chap. 28)

169. Answer: B

Patients with multiple failed trials are more likely to respond to clozapine than other agents. (Chap. 37)

170. Answer: E

St. John's wort has been used primarily to treat depression but has also been studied in other disorders. (Chap. 25)

171. Answer: A

Nicotinic receptors bind acetylcholine; they also bind nicotine. The other answer options are muscarinic receptor agonists. (Chap. 2)

172. Answer: B

Tics wax and wane in severity; this complicates prescribing, since improvement may be unrelated to medication use. (Chap. 36)

173. Answer: C

Having a child or adolescent's assent helps engagement and the treatment process. Informed consent is an ongoing process. (Chap. 27)

174. Answer: C

Separation anxiety disorder, along with specific phobia, tends to precede generalized anxiety disorder, social phobia, and then obsessive-compulsive disorder. (Chap. 34)

175. Answer: B

Adolescent patients with comorbid personality disorders showed a poorer response to a course of ECT in this study. ECT is not indicated for ODD and autism. (Chap. 26)

176. Answer: C

Trazodone is one of the most sedating antidepressant medications and is commonly used for sleep induction. (Chap. 46)

177. Answer: C

Steady-state concentration of a drug describes the equilibrium between the amount of drug ingested and amount of drug eliminated. (Chap. 3)

178. Answer: D

STAR*D did not find any difference in response among serotonin transporter variants. (Chap. 6)

179. Answer: B

Bupropion is FDA-approved for smoking cessation and depression in adults. (Chap. 21)

180. Answer: D

20% of children with Tourette's disorder continue to experience at least a moderate level of impairment in global functioning by age 20. (Chap. 12)

181. Answer: A

Melatonin has been shown to be effective for initial insomnia in patients with ADHD. (Chap. 24)

182. Answer: B

Stimulation of beta and alpha-1 receptors reduces functioning in the prefrontal cortex. Conversely, stimulation of alpha-2 receptors enhances functioning in the prefrontal cortex. (Chap. 11)

183. Answer: C

Pharmaceutical industry and academic relationships can pose significant conflicts of interest that need to be managed but are not inherently unethical. (Chap. 53)

184. Answer: E

Vital signs and an EKG should be obtained before initiating clomipramine and during treatment. (Chap. 35)

185.   Answer: C

A 54% response rate to psychostimulants for children with ADHD and intellectual disability is below the rate of 77% cited for typically developing children. (Chap. 42)

186.   Answer: B

Federal regulations require that two methadone-free rehabilitations are tried before methadone is prescribed in youths under 18. (Chap. 41)

187.   Answer: B

Combining monoamine oxidase inhibitors (MAOIs) with dextromethorphan (and meperidine) may result in serotonin syndrome and may also lead to complications from respiratory depression, including death. (Chap. 21)

188.   Answer: B

The MeCP2 gene encodes X-linked methyl-CpG-binding protein 2, which has been identified as the cause of the majority of cases of Rett's disorder. (Chap. 38)

189.   Answer: D

The presence of anxiety does not appear to decrease responsiveness to stimulant treatment. (Chap. 34)

190.   Answer: A

Schizophrenia is not associated specifically with childhood anxiety disorders, although patients with schizophrenia can have a range of childhood difficulties. (Chap. 34)

191.   Answer: D

Clomipramine has been shown to be efficacious in OCD. (Chap. 32)

192.   Answer: C

Short-term trials indicate that cognitive behavioral therapy is most effective, including superiority to IPT; however, at the 1-year follow-up, IPT and CBT were equal. (Chap. 40)

193.   Answer: C

Youths with EOSS are less likely to spontaneously report positive symptoms compared with adults. (Chap. 37)

194.   Answer: D

Therapeutic misconception in research refers to the notion that subjects believe their personal best interests will be served, even though the research objectives are paramount. This happens even when informed consent is thorough. (Chap. 52)

195.   Answer: A

SSRIs can cause hidrosis (increased perspiration) rather than anhidrosis. Bleeding is a concern that is especially relevant for patients undergoing surgical procedures or taking aspirin or nonsteroidal anti-inflammatory drugs. (Chap. 20)

196.   Answer: C

Chlorpromazine was first used as a tranquilizer and later as an antipsychotic in the 1950s. (Chap. 23)

197.   Answer: B

The half-life of clonidine in adults is 12 to 16 hours; it is 8 to 12 hours in children. (Chap. 19)

198.   Answer: C

Multiple daily doses have been recommended to minimize sedation and withdrawal and to maximize effect in comparison to a single large dose; this holds true even for benzodiazepines with relatively long half-lives. (Chap. 24)

199.   Answer: C

The effect of benzodiazepines is mediated by their action on $GABA_A$ receptors. (Chap. 46)

200.   Answer: C

Substance-use treatment, STD treatment, and birth control can be initiated with a minor's consent in a number of states. (Chap. 52)

Test 5 Questions

1. **Which antipsychotic has been associated with myocarditis?**

   A. Risperidone

   B. Olanzapine

   C. Quetiapine

   D. Ziprasidone

   E. Clozapine

2. **A psychiatrist treats a child with a selective serotonin reuptake inhibitor (SSRI) for anxiety and the child responds well. When should the psychiatrist consider tapering and discontinuing the SSRI?**

   A. After 2 months

   B. After 4 months

   C. After 1 year

   D. Lifelong treatment is indicated.

3. **Frontal gray matter volume peaks at about what age?**

   A. 10 years

   B. 16 years

   C. 22 years

   D. 34 years

4. **Which of the following statements is true?**

   A. When comparing U.S. studies and non-U.S. studies, the prevalence of ADHD is higher in non-U.S. studies.

   B. When comparing U.S. studies and non-U.S. studies, the prevalence of ADHD is higher in U.S. studies.

   C. When comparing U.S. studies and non-U.S. studies, the prevalence of ADHD is the same in U.S. and non-U.S. studies.

   D. U.S. and non-U.S. studies cannot be compared because of differing criteria used for ADHD.

5. **The American Academy of Child and Adolescent Psychiatry (AACAP) has made available free of charge which of the following?**

   A. Practice parameters

   B. The AACAP journal

   C. Samples of pharmaceuticals to indigent populations

   D. Toll-free line for consultations to community pediatricians

6. **Elevated depression scores during childhood and adolescence have a predictive value for what in later childhood, adolescence, and adulthood?**

   A. Depression

   B. Obesity

   C. Multiple suicide attempts

   D. Psychostimulant abuse

7. **In a large trial of 334 youths aged 12 to 18 who had depression resistant to SSRI treatment, switching to venlafaxine compared to switching to another SSRI was:**

   A. More efficacious

   B. Less efficacious

   C. Equivalent in efficacy

   D. Not efficacious at all

8. **Which of the following statements is FALSE regarding the Pre-school ADHD Treatment Study (PATS)?**

   A. In the first phase of the study, parent training alone was used.

   B. Children responded well to parent training alone.

   C. A pharmacokinetic study as part of the protocol demonstrated that preschoolers metabolized methylphenidate more slowly than school-age children.

   D. The effect sizes for parent and teacher ratings were smaller than that found for older children.

9. **What has been found regarding the effect of methylphenidate (MPH) in children with pervasive developmental disorders (PDDs) and hyperactivity in comparison with typically developing children with ADHD?**

    A. MPH has no beneficial effects for children with PDDs.

    B. MPH is more efficacious, with a decreased incidence of adverse events.

    C. MPH is equally efficacious, with the equal incidence of adverse events.

    D. MPH is less efficacious and associated with more frequent adverse events.

10. **Which of the following agents acts centrally as a serotonin and norepinephrine transporter blocker?**

    A. Metoclopramide

    B. Ondansetron

    C. Orlistat

    D. Sibutramine

11. **Which of the following four optical isomers of methylphenidate shows the greatest reuptake inhibition of dopamine and norepinephrine?**

    A. D-threo

    B. L-threo

    C. D-erythro

    D. L-erythro

12. **Which cytochrome P450 enzymes are most important for the clearance of antipsychotics?**

    A. 3A4, 2D6, 1A1

    B. 3A4, 2D6, 1A2

    C. 3A4, 2D6, 2B6

    D. 2D6, 1A2, 3A5

Match the following drugs that have been used or studied in tic disorders with the correct answer option.

13. **Nicotine**

14. **Botulinum**

15. **Intravenous immunoglobulin**

16. **Baclofen**

17. **Flutamide**

18. **Ondansetron**

19. **Levetiracetam**

20. **Topiramate**

21. **Mecamylamine**

    A. Decreased release of acetylcholine

    B. $GABA_B$ receptor agonist

    C. Available as chewing gum or a patch

    D. Nicotine antagonist

    E. Autoimmune response

    F. Enhances inhibitory effects of GABA at $GABA_A$

    G. Androgen receptor blocker

    H. Selective serotonin receptor antagonist

    I. Enhances GABA and blocks glutamate

The following questions concern an adult study by Harrigan and colleagues examining the QT prolongation of six commonly prescribed antipsychotics. Match the QT prolongation over baseline with the antipsychotic(s).

22. **30 milliseconds**

23. **15 milliseconds**

24. **3 to 7 milliseconds**

25. **<2 milliseconds**

    A. Thioridazine

    B. Ziprasidone

    C. Risperidone, haloperidol, and quetiapine

    D. Olanzapine

26. **Fetal exposure to valproate is associated with an increased rate of:**

    A. Atrial septal defects

    B. Neural tube defects

    C. Ebstein's anomaly

    D. Developmental delay

    E. Intellectual disability

27. The half-life of lamotrigine in children aged 5 to 11 years is 7 hours, but in combination with divalproex, the half-life increases to:

    A. 12 hours

    B. 26 hours

    C. 34 hours

    D. 66 hours

28. Which area of the brain has been implicated in the interpretation of the actions, intentions, and psychological dispositions of others through an analysis of biological-motion cues?

    A. Lateral fusiform gyrus

    B. Amygdala

    C. Orbitofrontal cortex

    D. Superior temporal sulcus

29. Which of the following agents has been used for neuropathic pain in children?

    A. Gabapentin

    B. Sertraline

    C. Carbamazepine

    D. Mirtazapine

30. Which of the following is LEAST likely to affect treatment recommendations?

    A. A family's attitudes and cultural beliefs regarding psychiatric illness

    B. The level of family dysfunction

    C. A child's co-occurring illnesses

    D. The cost of medications

    E. The birth order of the patient

31. Which of the following statements is most accurate?

    A. Combining a second-generation antipsychotic (SGA) with a mood stabilizer doubles the rate of weight gain.

    B. Combining an SGA with a stimulant attenuates the SGA associated weight gain.

    C. Combining an SGA with a mood stabilizer seems to be associated with less weight gain than with mood stabilizer monotherapy.

    D. Combining an SGA and a stimulant does not seem to attenuate SGA associated weight gain.

32. Which of the following medications is FDA-approved for pediatric enuresis?

    A. Propantheline

    B. Imipramine

    C. Oxybutynin

    D. Amitriptyline

33. Which of the following monoamine oxidase inhibitors (MAOIs) is considered the most sedating?

    A. Selegiline

    B. Phenelzine

    C. Tranylcypromine

    D. Isocarboxazid

34. Schizophrenia affects which percentage of the population?

    A. 1%

    B. 2%

    C. 5%

    D. 8%

35. Which serotonin receptor subtype has been extensively studied in schizophrenia?

    A. $5\text{-}HT_{1a}$

    B. $5\text{-}HT_{1d}$

    C. $5\text{-}HT_{2a}$

    D. $5\text{-}HT_{3}$

36. Which of the following would be considered first-line treatment for a pregnant, opiate-addicted teenager?

    A. Clonidine

    B. L-alpha acetylmethadol (LAAM)

    C. Methadone

    D. Naloxone

37. A meta-analysis examining neonates exposed to selective serotonin reuptake inhibitors (SSRIs) in the late third trimester through delivery found that 30% experience which of the following symptoms?

    A. Jitteriness

    B. Respiratory difficulties

    C. Irritability

    D. All of the above

38. The risk of serious and possibly fatal dermatologic reactions to carbamazepine increases in patients of which race?

    A. Caucasian

    B. African-American

    C. Hispanic

    D. Chinese

    E. Native American

39. What is the mechanism of action of diphenhydramine or hydroxyzine?

    A. Blockade of alpha1$_a$ receptors

    B. Blockade of H1 receptors

    C. Blockade of 5-HT2$_a$ receptors

    D. Blockade of orexin receptors

40. Which type of bipolar disorder requires the presence of at least one major depressive episode and one hypomanic episode?

    A. Bipolar I disorder

    B. Bipolar II disorder

    C. Cyclothymic disorder

    D. Bipolar disorder NOS

41. Childhood disintegrative disorder has had multiple prior names, including all of the following EXCEPT:

    A. Heller's syndrome

    B. Dementia praecox

    C. Dementia infantilis

    D. Disintegrative psychosis

42. A recent meta-analysis of randomized clinical trials for youths with major depressive disorder treated with selective serotonin reuptake inhibitors (SSRIs) as a class versus placebo resulted in which number needed to treat (NNT)?

    A. 2

    B. 4

    C. 10

    D. 15

43. Which of the following is an antihistaminic, 5-HT antagonist that has shown utility in reducing traumatic nightmares in a small number of studies?

    A. Hydroxyzine

    B. Diphenhydramine

    C. Nortriptyline

    D. Cyproheptadine

44. Which TWO of the following answer options are clinician-rated measurements for assessing symptom severity in non-OCD pediatric anxiety disorders?

    A. Hamilton Anxiety Rating Scale (HAM-A)

    B. Pediatric Anxiety Rating Scale (PARS)

    C. Spence Children's Anxiety Scale (SCAS)

    D. Multidimensional Anxiety Scale for Children (MASC)

45. Which of the following is the most abundant amino acid in the central nervous system (CNS)?

    A. Lysine

    B. Tyrosine

    C. Glutamate

    D. Tryptophan

46. Which neurotransmitter is used by interneurons for the inhibitory control of glutamatergic pathways?

    A. Dopamine

    B. Serotonin

    C. Glutamate

    D. GABA

47. All the following medications increase lithium levels EXCEPT:

    A. Ibuprofen

    B. Fluoxetine

    C. Ampicillin

    D. Lorazepam

    E. Lisinopril

48. What is the estimated rate of response to electro-convulsive therapy (ECT) in adults with major depression?
    A. 20%
    B. 40%
    C. 70%
    D. 90%

49. What effect does carbamazepine have on lamotrigine blood levels?
    A. Increases plasma lamotrigine by 25%
    B. Increases plasma lamotrigine by 50%
    C. Decreases plasma lamotrigine by 25%
    D. Decreases plasma lamotrigine by 50%
    E. No effect

50. Which of the following statements is accurate?
    A. Many tics are under partial voluntary control.
    B. Tics are under voluntary control.
    C. Tics are involuntary.
    D. Tics are most severe after the age of 20.

51. Trauma exposure occurs in what proportion of children?
    A. One-tenth
    B. One-fifth
    C. Two-thirds
    D. All children

52. For youths with early-onset schizophrenia spectrum disorders (EOSS), the use of marijuana has been associated with what feature?
    A. Delayed onset
    B. Earlier onset
    C. Decreased comorbid anxiety
    D. Increased comorbid anxiety

53. What percentage of children with a diagnosed anxiety disorder have some type of psychopathology in adulthood?
    A. 2.5%
    B. 25%
    C. 35%
    D. 50%

54. What possible contaminant might be found in fish oil capsules that would be of particular concern for children and pregnant women?
    A. Copper
    B. Lead
    C. Gold
    D. Arsenic
    E. Mercury

55. Amnestic deficits associated with electroconvulsive therapy (ECT) are greater for which types of memories?
    A. Knowledge about the world
    B. Knowledge about the self
    C. Recent events
    D. A and C

56. Alcohol has a "biphasic" effect on sleep architecture due to which of the following?
    A. Increasing REM sleep initially and then suppressing it later in the night
    B. Suppressing REM sleep initially, which results in a REM rebound as alcohol levels drop
    C. Decreasing slow-wave sleep initially and then increasing slow-wave sleep as alcohol levels drop
    D. Increasing slow-wave sleep initially and then decreasing slow-wave sleep as alcohol levels drop
    E. B and C

57. Approximately what percentage of patients with attention-deficit/hyperactivity disorder (ADHD) respond to the first stimulant selected?
    A. 33%
    B. 50%
    C. 67%
    D. 95%

58. Which chemical process leads to the uncoiling of chromatin at a particular gene site, allowing DNA to be transcribed?
    A. Histone acetylation
    B. Triplet repeats
    C. DNA methylation
    D. Translation

59. Which of the following was once touted as a cure for autism, but considerable evidence now shows it is of no benefit?

    A. St. John's wort

    B. Kava

    C. Secretin

    D. S-adenosyl methionine

60. Which of the following is a potential clinical manifestation of prolactin elevation?

    A. Gynecomastia

    B. Galactorrhea

    C. Menstrual irregularities

    D. All of the above

61. Symptom rating scales are often used in clinical trials. Which of the following is another method to measure response to treatment?

    A. Calling the child's coach

    B. Asking the child's sibling

    C. Communicating with the probation officer

    D. Counting discrete events

62. What is the mechanism of action of methylphenidate?

    A. Blocks the dopamine transporter, increasing dopamine in synapse and extracellular space

    B. Blocks norepinephrine reuptake, increasing norepinephrine in synapse and extracellular space

    C. A and B

    D. None of the above

63. A characteristic polysomnographic finding in patients on selective serotonin reuptake inhibitors (SSRIs) has been given the nickname of "Prozac eyes" due to which observed phenomenon?

    A. Increased REM density

    B. Decreased REM density

    C. Absence of REM activity

    D. Increased slow-wave sleep

64. According to National Ambulatory Medical Care Survey data, approximately 50% of visits for ADHD in 1989 resulted in the prescription of a stimulant. What is that percentage today?

    A. <25%

    B. 25% to 50%

    C. 50% to 75%

    D. >75%

65. The consideration of what attribute in a pharmacological agent to address insomnia will minimize the "morning hangover" or persistent grogginess effect?

    A. Receptor profile

    B. Half-life

    C. Suppression of REM sleep

    D. Effect on slow-wave sleep

66. Separating rat pups from their mothers has been reported to lead to which of the following phenomena later in life?

    A. Greater anxiety levels

    B. Increased consumption and response to alcohol

    C. Increased consumption and response to psychostimulants

    D. All of the above

67. A 17-year-old boy develops acne and gains 8 lbs after beginning lithium 8 weeks ago. Which is an associated side effect of lithium treatment?

    A. Acne

    B. Weight gain

    C. Both acne and weight gain

    D. None of the above

68. What is the half-life of guanfacine (immediate-release formulation) in adults and children?

    A. 50 hours in adults and 24 hours in children

    B. 8 hours in adults and 4 hours in children

    C. 13 hours in adults and 36 hours in children

    D. 17 hours in adults and 14 hours in children

69. Patients develop physiologic dependence from chronic benzodiazepine use within what general time frame?

    A. 1 to 2 weeks

    B. 2 weeks to 1 month

    C. 3 to 4 months

    D. 1 year

70. Which of the following is an agonist of the GABA$_B$ receptor?

    A. Lorazepam

    B. Baclofen

    C. Oxazepam

    D. Buspirone

71. What is the age range for the childhood onset of obsessive-compulsive disorder?

    A. 4 to 9 years

    B. 7 to 12 years

    C. 12 to 15 years

    D. >15 years

72. Paroxetine has FDA approval for what disorders in children?

    A. Major depressive disorder (MDD)

    B. Posttraumatic stress disorder (PTSD)

    C. Generalized anxiety disorder (GAD)

    D. Obsessive-compulsive disorder (OCD)

    E. None

73. Removal of acetylcholine from the neuronal synapse can be blocked by acetylcholinesterase inhibitors, which include:

    A. Pilocarpine

    B. Physostigmine

    C. Bethanechol

    D. Atropine

74. In children with a seizure disorder and attention-deficit/hyperactivity disorder (ADHD), which of the following statements is most accurate?

    A. Methylphenidate should never be used in seizure disorders.

    B. Methylphenidate has been shown to lower seizure threshold through controlled studies.

    C. Methylphenidate can be used when a child's seizures are controlled.

    D. Methylphenidate increases the risk of seizures in children with epileptiform discharges.

75. What is the optimal time after the last dose to measure serum valproate levels?

    A. 2 hours

    B. 6 hours

    C. 10 hours

    D. 12 hours

    E. 18 hours

76. What is the main mechanism of action of St. John's wort for depression?

    A. Serotonin reuptake inhibition

    B. Serotonin and norepinephrine reuptake inhibition

    C. Dopamine and serotonin agonism

    D. Alpha agonism

    E. The mechanism is unknown.

77. True or False. Pregabalin has been approved for the treatment of anxiety disorders in adults.

    A. True

    B. False

78. Which term describes how well a screening or diagnostic instrument actually measures what it is supposed to measure?

    A. Reliability

    B. Validity

    C. Sensitivity

    D. Specificity

79. The effect size for stimulants in the treatment of pediatric aggression is medium to large and closest to:

    A. 0.3

    B. 0.5

    C. 0.8

    D. 1.2

80. Clozapine blood levels should be greater than which concentration in patients who have failed multiple antipsychotic trials?

    A. 100 ng/dL

    B. 150 ng/dL

    C. 250 ng/dL

    D. 350 ng/dL

81. Which of the following is LEAST likely to be a relevant question for a clinical trial?

    A. Is the treatment effective in inducing full recovery from the disorder?

    B. Is long-term treatment needed to prevent relapse or maintain recovery?

    C. Is the treatment likely to be used by a given family?

    D. How does the treatment compare with alternative psychopharmacological or psychosocial treatments?

    E. Is the treatment effective across different clinical settings, in usual practice?

82. Which TWO factors have been found to be modestly associated with a worse response to psychostimulants in children?

    A. Lower IQ

    B. Higher frequency of disruptive behaviors

    C. Lower mental age

    D. Presence of comorbid conduct disorder

83. Clomipramine acts at which main neurotransmitter system(s)?

    A. Serotonin

    B. Serotonin and norepinephrine

    C. Norepinephrine

    D. Serotonin, norepinephrine, dopamine

84. Which of the following best captures the risk of suicidal thinking or behaviors with SSRIs compared to placebo?

    A. 1% compared to 0.5%

    B. 4% compared to 2%

    C. 6% compared to 2%

    D. 8% compared to 2%

85. Which of the following physiological systems is involved in trauma?

    A. Neuroendocrine

    B. Immune

    C. Central nervous system

    D. All of the above

86. Approximately what percentage of children and adolescents who have dysthymic disorder will eventually meet criteria for major depressive disorder (MDD) in the future?

    A. 70%

    B. 50%

    C. 35%

    D. 15%

87. When should an antipsychotic be discontinued?

    A. QTc of >500 msec confirmed by manual reading

    B. Relative increase from baseline QTc of >60 msec

    C. QTc of >450 msec confirmed by manual reading

    D. A and B

    E. B and C

88. When mood improvements were observed in patients treated with the tuberculosis drug iproniazid, the mood-enhancing quality of which class of medications was serendipitously discovered?

    A. Tricyclic antidepressants (TCAs)

    B. Monoamine oxidase inhibitors (MAOIs)

    C. Selective serotonin reuptake inhibitors (SSRIs)

    D. First-generation antipsychotics

89. Why is the use of an anticholinergic agent such as atropine or glycopyrrolate recommended during electroconvulsive therapy (ECT)?

    A. To minimize excessive vagal activity

    B. To minimize excessive sympathetic outflow

    C. To increase secretions in the bronchial airways

    D. To reduce confusion after treatment

Match each of the following drug compounds with its principal serotonin receptor type.

90. Buspirone

91. LSD

92. Psilocybin

93. Sumatriptan

    A. 5-HT_{1A}

    B. 5-HT_{2A}

    C. 5-HT_{1D}

Match the dopaminergic neuronal pathway with its associated behavior (multiple answers possible).

94. Ventral tegmental area to limbic structures

95. Ventral tegmental area to cortex

96. Hypothalamus to the pituitary gland

    A. Inhibit the production and release of prolactin

    B. Involved in appetitive and reward behavior

    C. Play a role in the fine-tuning of cortical neurons—that is, improving signal-to-noise ratio

    D. Involved in the development of addiction to drugs such as cocaine, nicotine, and opiates

97. Clinical studies of selective serotonin reuptake inhibitors (SSRIs) in anorexia nervosa have shown which of the following?

    A. Severely malnourished patients on SSRIs improve their obsessionality.

    B. Severely malnourished patients do no better on SSRIs.

    C. Severely malnourished patients improve their depressive symptoms.

    D. Severely malnourished patients on SSRIs have better weight gain.

98. Which set of agents has the least CYP450 inhibition?

    A. Citalopram, escitalopram, paroxetine, sertraline, venlafaxine

    B. Citalopram, escitalopram, fluoxetine, sertraline, venlafaxine

    C. Citalopram, escitalopram, paroxetine, sertraline, fluoxetine

    D. Escitalopram, paroxetine, fluoxetine, sertraline, venlafaxine

99. Levels of which benzodiazepine are increased by co-administration of fluoxetine?

    A. Lorazepam

    B. Clonazepam

    C. Temazepam

    D. Midazolam

100. Which of the following is considered a uridine diphosphate glucuronosyltransferase (UGT)-based drug–drug interaction?

    A. Risperidone and fluoxetine

    B. Aripiprazole and fluoxetine

    C. Carbamazepine with itself

    D. Lamotrigine and valproic acid

101. In what decade was transcranial magnetic stimulation (TMS) first used?

    A. 1920s

    B. 1950s

    C. 1980s

    D. 2000s

102. Which of the following options properly lists the neuromodulatory and neurotransmitter systems implicated in Tourette's disorder?

    A. Dopamine, glutamate, serotonin

    B. Dopamine, brain-derived neurotrophic factor, serotonin

    C. Dopamine, glutamate, GABA, endogenous opioids, norepinephrine, serotonin

    D. Dopamine, serotonin, norepinephrine

103. A child does not respond to a second SSRI after a first trial. You should most consider a switch to:

    A. Clomipramine

    B. Haloperidol

    C. Risperidone

    D. Another SSRI

104. The pharmacokinetic term *clearance* describes what process?

    A. Absorption

    B. Elimination

    C. Distribution

    D. Bioavailability

105. After what period in gestation has fetal-placental circulation been established?

    A. Upon conception

    B. After 20 days

    C. After 50 days

    D. After the first trimester

106. A child with anorexia nervosa presents with depression. Which is the most likely explanation?

    A. There is a family history of mood disorders.

    B. The patient is using food restriction as a method to cope with dysphoria.

    C. Starvation

    D. The child is using depression as an excuse for poor eating.

107. True or False. Prepubertal children who present with major depressive disorder have a decreased risk for subsequently developing bipolar disorder.

    A. True

    B. False

108. What is a sequential multiple assignment randomized trial (SMART)?

    A. Subjects are randomized to a particular intervention with sequential clinician raters.

    B. Subjects are randomized to a particular intervention with change in assignment after a specified time.

    C. Subjects are randomized to a particular intervention with a sequential shift in primary outcome measures.

    D. Subjects are randomized to a particular intervention and are later randomized to a second treatment or control condition depending on the response to the first treatment.

109. After what age does the total brain volume show minimal increase?

    A. 2 years

    B. 5 years

    C. 15 years

    D. 20 years

For the following questions, match the instrument with its corresponding description.

110. Eating Disorder Examination (EDE)

111. Structured Interview for Anorexia and Bulimia Nervosa (SIAB)

112. Eating Disorder Inventory (EDI-3)

113. Eating Attitudes Test (EAT)

    A. Self-report questionnaire on disordered eating (26 items)

    B. Useful in assessing areas of psychopathology and interpersonal problems (91 items)

    C. A semi-structured, clinician-administered interview that focuses on the present state of patients (62 items)

    D. Assesses family interaction and pathology in addition to core eating disorder psychopathology (87 items)

114. Continuing medical education (CME) presentations:

    A. Represent an inherent conflict of interest

    B. Serve to maintain, develop, and increase the knowledge, skills, and professional performance of physicians

    C. Have come under increasing regulatory scrutiny and will be banned under the sunset clause of President Obama's American Recovery and Reinvestment Act

    D. Are frequently delivered by laypersons

115. In every 100 youths treated with selective serotonin reuptake inhibitors (SSRIs), there is an increase of how many spontaneously reported adverse events of suicidality?

    A. 2 or 3

    B. 3 to 5

    C. 5 to 7

    D. 7 to 9

116. Concomitant use of which of the following medications could decrease the effectiveness of electroconvulsive therapy (ECT)?

    A. Benzodiazepines

    B. Topiramate

    C. Gabapentin

    D. All of the above

117. The risk for extrapyramidal symptoms with antipsychotics, especially parkinsonian symptoms, is primarily related to:

    A. Anticholinergic properties

    B. Dopamine D2 receptor antagonism

    C. Dopamine D4 receptor antagonism

    D. 5-HT2$_a$ reuptake inhibition

118. Which term describes the clinical or research measure that generates many gradations in the variable of interest?

    A. Continuous measure

    B. Categorical measure

    C. Dimensional measure

    D. A and C

119. Which of the following has been reported as attributable to atomoxetine?

    A. Osteosarcoma

    B. Psoriasis

    C. Liver injury

    D. Pulmonary embolism

120. A survey of the literature on the prevalence of schizophrenia in patients with intellectual disability found what average rate?

    A. 0.5%

    B. 1%

    C. 2%

    D. 3%

121. Specific phobias in children generally cluster into three subtypes. Which of the following is NOT one of the subtypes?

    A. Animal phobias

    B. Blood/injection/injury phobias

    C. Environmental/situational phobias

    D. Movement phobias

122. The brain areas involved in obsessive-compulsive disorder (OCD) are the:

    A. Prefrontal-subcortical circuits

    B. Frontal-cerebellar circuits

    C. Frontal-subcortical circuits

    D. Prefrontal-limbic circuits

123. The most serious adverse effect for children ingesting clonidine at 0.3 mg or above is:

    A. Lightheadedness

    B. Dizziness

    C. Syncope

    D. Coma

124. The Food and Drug Administration (FDA) labeling for stimulants includes a warning that:

    A. Patients with poor eating habits should not use stimulants.

    B. Patients with heart defects might be at particular risk for sudden death, and stimulants should not ordinarily be used.

    C. Patients with narcolepsy should not ordinarily be prescribed stimulants.

    D. Patients with history of substance use should not be prescribed stimulants.

125. Mood stabilizers can be divided into two classes: the traditional agents and the newer or "novel" agents. The novel agents include all the following EXCEPT:

    A. Lamotrigine

    B. Oxcarbazepine

    C. Topiramate

    D. Pregabalin

    E. Carbamazepine

126. Which of the following approaches was found useful in the treatment of bulimia nervosa or bulimia nervosa-like symptoms in eating disorder, not otherwise specified (ED NOS)?

    A. Pairing two adolescents who are recovering and stipulating text message check-in

    B. One group session and then providing list of vetted Internet sites that address eating disorders

    C. Group sessions over 12 weeks through Facebook interaction

    D. Internet sessions with patient along with peer and parent support through message boards

127. Which of these is NOT a rating scale?

    A. The Johnson-Smith Dyskinesia Scale

    B. The Simpson-Angus Scale for Parkinsonian Side Effects

    C. The Barnes Akathisia Scale

    D. The Abnormal Involuntary Movement Scale

128. The U.S. government established what agency in 1998 to explore complementary and alternative medicine practices in the context of rigorous science?

    A. The Complementary Medicine Association (CMS)

    B. The National Center for Complementary and Alternative Medicine (NCCAM)

    C. The National Institutes of Health

    D. The National Institute of Mental Health

129. What protein is commonly involved in drug transport during absorption and can be affected by substrate, inducer, and inhibitor drugs?

    A. Cyclic adenosine monophosphate

    B. Inositol

    C. P-glycoprotein

    D. Brain-derived neurotrophic factor

130. According to studies, what is the range of placebo response in pediatric obsessive-compulsive disorder (OCD)?

    A. 10% to 25%

    B. 25% to 35%

    C. >50%

    D. >75%

131. Which of the following statements is accurate about substance use?

    A. Onset of drinking before the age of 14 is likely to lead to higher levels of dependence and abuse than drinking that begins in later adolescence or adulthood.

    B. Pediatric substance use has low heritability.

    C. There are no biochemical differences between those who have earlier rather than later onset of substance use.

    D. Risky sexual behavior is not correlated with substance use.

132. Which of the following is a reason antipsychotics are limited in their utility for attention-deficit/hyperactivity disorder (ADHD)?

    A. They are ineffective.

    B. The side-effect profile

    C. There are no studies of antipsychotics in ADHD.

    D. Children have trouble swallowing available formulations.

133. What is the primary site of absorption of most benzodiazepines?

    A. Sublingual duct

    B. Submandibular duct

    C. Gastrointestinal tract

    D. Liver

134. Which term describes the probability that a child identified by a screening instrument as having a disorder or symptom actually does have it?

    A. Face validity

    B. Content validity

    C. Positive predictive power

    D. Negative predictive power

135. Which of the following words describes the period when the synaptic circuitry of a given brain region becomes stabilized in a functionally optimized conformation?

    A. Diversification

    B. Neuronal migration

    C. Maturation

    D. Apoptosis

    E. Critical period

136. The COBY (Course of Bipolar Illness in Youth) study found that youths with bipolar disorder had which attributes in comparison to adults with bipolar disorder?

    A. Youths with bipolar disorder spent more time symptomatic.

    B. Youths with bipolar disorder had greater cycling episodes.

    C. Youths with bipolar disorder had greater mixed episodes.

    D. All of the above

137. Global reduction in brain volume, which has been found in subjects with attention-deficit/hyperactivity disorder (ADHD), occurs in:

    A. Gray matter only

    B. White matter only

    C. Both gray and white matter

    D. None of the above

138. Which of the following disorders is LEAST likely to be treated with an alpha agonist?

    A. Posttraumatic stress disorder

    B. Attention-deficit/hyperactivity disorder

    C. Oppositional defiant disorder

    D. Conduct disorder

    E. Major depressive disorder

139. A child with obsessive-compulsive disorder (OCD) has partially responded to a second selective serotonin reuptake inhibitor (SSRI) trial. Which of the following would be a reasonable augmentation strategy?

    A. Guanfacine

    B. Risperidone

    C. Lithium

    D. Bupropion

140. Which of the following definitions best describes epigenetics?

    A. Changes in gene expression caused by mechanisms other than changes in the DNA sequence

    B. Changes in gene expression caused by changes in the DNA sequence

    C. Changes in environment causing changes in the DNA sequence

    D. B and C

141. The trial phase also known as a "microdosing study" that explores whether a drug behaves in humans as expected from preclinical studies is known as:

    A. Phase 0

    B. Phase I

    C. Phase II

    D. Phase III

    E. Phase IV

142. In pharmacodynamic studies, what is the role of genetic studies?

    A. They focus on cytochrome P450 polymorphisms.

    B. They focus on individual patient differences to drug response.

    C. They focus on genetic variations affecting the sites of drug action.

    D. They focus on drug development related to allelic variations.

143. Which agent was considered the first "atypical" antipsychotic?

    A. Clozapine

    B. Risperidone

    C. Olanzapine

    D. Quetiapine

    E. Perphenazine

144. You are treating a child with obsessive-compulsive disorder (OCD) who fails to respond to his first medication trial, an SSRI prescribed at a maximum dose for an adequate length of time. What is your next strategy?

    A. Clomipramine

    B. Quetiapine

    C. Risperidone

    D. Another SSRI

    E. Mirtazapine

145. Children tend to exhibit a relatively abrupt increase in panic attacks around which developmental stage?

    A. Oedipal period

    B. Latency

    C. Puberty

    D. Late adolescence

146. Early childhood assessments are generally best completed in the course of:

  A. One extended session

  B. Multiple visits

  C. A pediatrician's visit

  D. A school assessment

147. There has been an increase over the past two decades in the rate of psychotropic prescriptions to preschoolers, with approximately 2% of preschoolers currently receiving psychotropic prescriptions in a given year. All drug classes have shown increases. What is the most common drug class responsible for this increase?

  A. Stimulants

  B. Alpha agonists

  C. Antipsychotics

  D. Antidepressants

148. What have systematic studies of the effect of clonidine on electrocardiograms (ECG) found?

  A. Prolonged QTc

  B. No consistent effects on ECG

  C. Left ventricular hypertrophy

  D. Prolonged PR interval

  E. Sinus tachycardia

149. Which of the following statements best describes the concept of external validity in clinical research?

  A. The effectiveness of an intervention under usual conditions

  B. The effectiveness of an intervention under ideal conditions

  C. The extent to which results can be generalized to clinical populations

  D. The extent to which a study is methodologically sound

150. Which TWO factors affect drug distribution in the body?

  A. Body fat

  B. Gastric emptying time

  C. Total body water

  D. Drug polarity

151. When tapering clonidine, which of the following statements is FALSE?

  A. Clonidine can be abruptly discontinued if it has been used for less than a week.

  B. Clonidine should be tapered by 0.05 mg daily if it has been used 1 to 4 weeks.

  C. Clonidine should be tapered by 0.05 mg every 3 days if it has been used more than 4 weeks.

  D. Clonidine can be abruptly discontinued if it has been used to treat ADHD rather than hypertension.

152. There are no randomized clinical trials for the management of pediatric behavioral emergencies. From clinical experience all of the following agents are used EXCEPT:

  A. Droperidol

  B. Haloperidol

  C. Diphenhydramine

  D. Midazolam

153. Trials of ziprasidone for the treatment of early-onset schizophrenia spectrum disorders (EOSS) indicate what general level of efficacy?

  A. Highly effective

  B. Moderately effective

  C. Mildly effective

  D. Not effective

154. Which of the following is an accurate statement about zolpidem, zaleplon, and eszopiclone?

  A. They have a long onset of action.

  B. They have little effect on sleep architecture.

  C. They have a long half-life.

  D. Tolerance develops within three days.

155. One large double-blind study of youth with generalized anxiety disorder, separation anxiety, and social phobia found what effect size for sertraline?

  A. 0.25

  B. 0.45

  C. 1.05

  D. 3.45

156. All of the following tricyclic antidepressants have established therapeutic blood levels EXCEPT:

    A. Imipramine

    B. Amitriptyline

    C. Doxepin

    D. Clomipramine

157. Which of the following is a melatonin agonist?

    A. Eszopiclone

    B. Ramelteon

    C. Mirtazapine

    D. Hydroxyzine

158. Pharmacokinetics can be defined simply as:

    A. What the body does to the drug

    B. What the drug does to the body

    C. Both of the above

    D. None of the above

159. Which two anxiety disorders are defined under "Disorders Usually First Diagnosed in Infancy and Childhood"?

    A. Attention-deficit/hyperactivity disorder and selective mutism

    B. Selective mutism and generalized anxiety disorder

    C. Separation anxiety disorder and selective mutism

    D. Oppositional defiant disorder and attention-deficit/hyperactivity disorder

160. In a patient with severe asthma or cystic fibrosis, which of the following would be potentially most medically problematic?

    A. Dysthymia

    B. Past sexual abuse

    C. Anxiety

    D. Attention-deficit/hyperactivity disorder

161. In the guidelines developed by the Child and Adolescent Bipolar Foundation (CABF) for bipolar I disorder, manic or mixed without psychosis, monotherapy with which of the following is recommended?

    A. Mood stabilizer

    B. Tricyclic antidepressant

    C. Atypical antipsychotic

    D. Alpha agonist

    E. A or C

162. Which of the following offers the most accurate description of intermittent explosive disorder?

    A. Failure to resist aggressive impulses resulting in serious assaultive acts or destruction of property in the face of limited provocation and usually accompanied by remorse

    B. Sudden, unpredictable acts of physical assault or property destruction triggered by minimal provocation

    C. Failure to resist aggressive impulses resulting in assaultive acts or destruction of property

    D. The defensive function of acting out that is triggered by small provocations that lead to unregulated feelings of narcissistic injury and aggressive behaviors

163. In the classification of medications by the FDA, which classification denotes findings of minimal adverse effects on the human fetus?

    A. B

    B. C

    C. D

    D. X

164. Escitalopram has FDA approval for what disorder(s)?

    A. Adolescent major depressive disorder

    B. Adolescent generalized anxiety disorder

    C. Adolescent PTSD

    D. A and B

    E. A, B, and C

165. Plasma steady-state concentration describes the equilibrium between which two factors?

    A. Amount of drug eliminated and the saturation of drug metabolism

    B. Amount of drug ingested and amount of drug eliminated

    C. Time required for the drug concentration to decrease by 50% and amount of drug eliminated

    D. None of the above

166. Absorption of a drug depends heavily on the route of entry. Which kind of administration produces the equivalent of 100% absorption?

    A. Oral

    B. Intravenous

    C. Transcutaneous

    D. Inhalant

167. Studies of adults and adolescents with attention-deficit/hyperactivity disorder (ADHD) comorbid with substance use have generally found that longitudinally:

    A. Symptoms of ADHD may improve but substance use remains the same.

    B. Symptoms of ADHD worsen with treatment, while substance use improves.

    C. Symptoms of both ADHD and substance use worsen.

    D. Symptoms of schizotypal disorder develop.

168. What does the Latin word "placebo" mean?

    A. "I shall deceive"

    B. "I shall placate"

    C. "I shall please"

    D. "I shall confound"

169. What is the estimated lifetime incidence of physical and sexual abuse for child and adolescent psychiatric inpatients?

    A. 15%

    B. 25%

    C. 45%

    D. 55%

170. In what decade were the monoamine oxidase inhibitors discovered to be effective in the treatment of depression?

    A. 1900s

    B. 1920s

    C. 1940s

    D. 1960s

171. Mutations in the melanocortin-4 receptor gene (MC4R), which in adult heterozygous carriers account for an excess of 15 to 30 kg of weight, occur approximately in what percentage of obese adults?

    A. 0.25%

    B. 1%

    C. 2%

    D. 6%

172. A recent review of the literature on naltrexone therapy to treat self-injurious behaviors concluded that what percentage of patients showed at least some benefit with the medication?

    A. 80%

    B. 60%

    C. 35%

    D. 15%

173. The risk of relapse is much higher in which population of pediatric patients who have been treated for major depressive disorder?

    A. Those with an initial positive response to fluoxetine

    B. Those who have not attained full remission

    C. Those who engage in concurrent cognitive behavioral therapy (CBT)

    D. None of the above

174. A random population sample of 572 families found about what percentage of children 17 months old were physically aggressive to peers, siblings, and adults?

    A. 5%

    B. 25%

    C. 45%

    D. 70%

175. Monoamine oxidase inhibitors (MAOIs) can contribute to a hypertensive crisis when combined with which of the following?

    A. Aged meats

    B. Cheeses

    C. Stimulants

    D. All of the above

176. In medication pharmacotherapy for tics, an appropriate expectation of treatment is:

    A. Tic elimination

    B. Tic prophylaxis

    C. Tic reduction

    D. Tic elimination and prophylaxis

177. Each of the following is a biochemical mechanism of CYP inhibition EXCEPT:

    A. Synergistic

    B. Competitive

    C. Mechanism-based

    D. Metabolite-intermediate-complex

178. Constipation is a potential adverse effect of all anticholinergic agents and which of the following medications?

    A. Divalproex

    B. Trazodone

    C. Imipramine

    D. All of the above

179. The target problems in medication treatment may or may not be consistent with the defining symptoms of the disorder. For which one of the following disorders would the target problems addressed by medication likely be consistent with the disorder's defining features?

    A. Autism

    B. Attention-deficit/hyperactivity disorder

    C. Somatization disorder

    D. Factitious disorder

    E. Gender identity disorder

180. A clinical intervention would be considered very effective with which number needed to treat (NNT)?

    A. 3

    B. 30

    C. 60

    D. 100

181. Melatonin is a hormone secreted by the pineal gland and binds to receptors in the:

    A. Amygdala

    B. Thalamus

    C. Hypothalamus

    D. Prefrontal cortex

    E. Substantia nigra

182. A 16-year-old girl has been using levonorgestrel (Norplant) for contraception and is treated for bipolar disorder with valproic acid. Another agent is added, and it leads to breakthrough bleeding. Which agent is likely responsible?

    A. Lorazepam

    B. Lamotrigine

    C. Bupropion

    D. Lithium

    E. Topiramate

183. All the following are mania-specific screening instruments EXCEPT:

    A. Parent Mood Disorder Questionnaire (MDQ)

    B. Parent General Behavior Inventory (Parent GBI)

    C. Child Behavior Checklist (CBCL)

    D. Child Mania Rating Scale (CMRS)

184. Which of the following brain regions regulates executive functioning?

    A. Inferior temporal cortex

    B. Posterior parietal association cortex

    C. Prefrontal cortex

    D. Basal ganglia

185. Which statement best captures the current question of under- and over-prescribing for attention-deficit/hyperactivity disorder (ADHD)?

    A. Stimulants are over-prescribed.

    B. Stimulants are under-prescribed.

    C. Stimulants are over-prescribed and alpha agonists are under-prescribed.

    D. There are areas of over-prescription and other areas of under-prescription.

186. **The Multimodal Treatment Study for ADHD (MTA) found which of the following?**

    A. Stimulants worsened anxiety.

    B. Combined behavioral and medication treatment yielded less improvement in anxious children.

    C. Children assigned to the behavioral therapy arm alone who were identified also as having anxiety showed a positive response to behavioral treatment on parent-reported measures of ADHD and anxious symptoms.

    D. Modafinil worsened anxiety.

187. **Which category of antidepressant medications does duloxetine occupy based on its mechanism of action?**

    A. Selective serotonin/norepinephrine reuptake inhibitors (SNRI)

    B. Selective serotonin reuptake inhibitor (SSRI)

    C. Tricyclic antidepressant (TCA)

    D. Exact mechanism of action unknown

188. **Which of the following second-generation antipsychotics should be considered as a second-line agent for the treatment of adolescents?**

    A. Risperidone

    B. Quetiapine

    C. Ziprasidone

    D. Aripiprazole

189. **A large study linking population health data, maternal health, and prenatal prescription records found that first-trimester exposure to which of the following medications increased the risk of congenital anomalies and cardiac defects?**

    A. Benzodiazepines

    B. Selective serotonin reuptake inhibitors (SSRIs)

    C. Co-administration of benzodiazepines and SSRIs

    D. None of the above

190. **Which of the following metabolic reactions compose phase II metabolism?**

    A. Oxidation

    B. Reduction

    C. Hydrolysis

    D. Conjugation

191. **Co-administration of bupropion with monoamine oxidase inhibitors (MAOIs) risks which of the following?**

    A. Seizures

    B. Hypertensive crisis

    C. QT prolongation

    D. A and B

192. **The risk of occurrence of schizophrenia spectrum disorders in families related to a patient diagnosed with childhood-onset schizophrenia compared with adult-onset schizophrenia appears to be:**

    A. Equivalent

    B. Lower

    C. Higher

    D. Significantly lower

193. **Which of the following is a non-benzodiazepine receptor agonists intended to address insomnia?**

    A. Zaleplon

    B. Diphenhydramine

    C. Eszopiclone

    D. A and C

194. **When a medication is being tested for a condition in which other treatments exist, what is the problem with using placebo for a clinical trial?**

    A. Patients may be randomized to an inferior treatment.

    B. Patients are more likely to agree to the study.

    C. Patients will have expectations about treatment based on prior treatments.

    D. The number of reported side effects during the trial is likely to be greater.

195. **The Child-Adolescent Anxiety Multimodal Study (CAMS), the largest pediatric anxiety study to date, demonstrated which of the following?**

    A. The combination of sertraline and CBT is superior to either alone.

    B. Sertraline was no more effective than placebo.

    C. CBT was no more effective than placebo.

    D. The placebo control group had a better outcome than the sertraline group.

196. Which of the following statements describes dysfunctional voiding?

    A. Chronic withholding of urine and stool

    B. Palpable stool within the abdomen

    C. Unaware of the need to void

    D. All of the above

197. All of the following tricyclic antidepressants are secondary amines EXCEPT:

    A. Nortriptyline

    B. Trimipramine

    C. Desipramine

    D. Protriptyline

198. Which of the following agents prevents the breakdown of acetaldehyde producing an aversive reaction when alcohol is consumed?

    A. Naltrexone

    B. Disulfiram

    C. Sibutramine

    D. Acamprosate

199. The cognitive effects of alpha-adrenergic receptor agonists, including enhanced working memory, attention, and delayed responding, are mediated primarily by:

    A. Presynaptic alpha-2a mechanisms

    B. Post-synaptic dopaminergic receptors

    C. Post-synaptic serotonergic receptors

    D. Post-synaptic alpha-2a mechanisms

200. When switching from an antipsychotic that is strongly anti-dopaminergic to one that is less tightly bound to or a partial agonist of the dopamine D2 receptor, all the following may occur EXCEPT:

    A. Agitation

    B. Hyperphagia

    C. Akathisia

    D. Withdrawal dyskinesia

    E. Psychosis

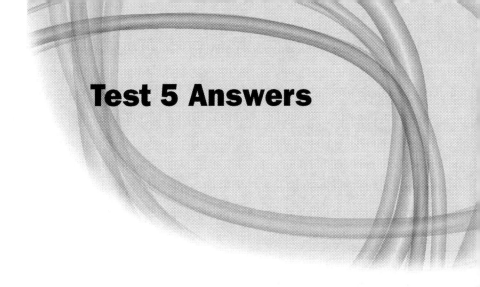

Test 5 Answers

1. Answer: E

Only clozapine has been associated with myocarditis. (Chap. 23)

2. Answer: C

Tapering and discontinuing an SSRI in pediatric anxiety often leads to high relapse rates if done prematurely. Waiting for a low stress period and a year (some say 6 months minimum) is advised. (Chap. 34)

3. Answer: A

Frontal gray matter volume peaks at about age 10 and then begins to thin; however, white matter volume continues to increase in the prefrontal region though all of childhood and into early adulthood. (Chap. 15)

4. Answer: C

When one compares U.S. studies and non-U.S. studies, the prevalence of ADHD is the same, especially when using DSM criteria. Prevalence estimates are 5% to 8%. (Chap. 31)

5. Answer: A

AACAP has made its practice parameters available free of charge; there are over 30 parameters. These are available at http://aacap.org/cs/root/member_information/practice_information/practice_parameters/practice_parameters. (Chap. 27)

6. Answer: B

Findings of multiple studies linking depression scores to subsequent weight gain are remarkably consistent. The duration of depression between childhood and adulthood also emerged as a predictor of adult BMI. (Chap. 16)

7. Answer: C

In the Treatment of SSRI-Resistant Depression in Adolescents (TORDIA) study, a switch to venlafaxine or another SSRI was equivalent in efficacy. There were more adverse effects in the group treated with venlafaxine. (Chap. 21)

8. Answer: B

All subjects started with parent training alone, but only 37 of 303 had a satisfactory response with parent training. The effect sizes were 0.35 and 0.43 respectively for parent and teacher ratings compared to effect sizes of 0.52 and 0.75 for older children in the MTA. (Chap. 18)

9. Answer: D

The study (RUPP Autism Network, 2005b) involved 72 children with PDDs with moderate to severe hyperactivity. It is efficacious but less so, and the dose-response curve is not as linear. (Chap. 38)

10. Answer: D

Sibutramine has FDA approval in obesity for patients >16 years of age. It likely functions as a weight-loss agent by reducing the threshold to satiety. (Chap. 40)

11. Answer: A

The standard preparation of methylphenidate has been the threo racemic mixture as it appears to be the CNS active form; of this racemic mixture, D-threo appears to be a more potent inhibitor of dopamine and norepinephrine reuptake. (Chap. 31)

12. Answer: B

The CYP enzymes 3A4, 2D6, and 1A2 are most important in antipsychotic metabolism. (Chap. 23)

13–21. Answers

13-C; 14-A; 15-E; 16-B; 17-G; 18-H; 19-F; 20-I; 21-D.

There are varying degrees of evidence for each of these potential anti-tic agents, studied based on their purported mechanisms of action, with open and/or closed trials showing some promise or no effect. Ondansetron and topiramate have been shown to be superior to placebo in relatively small trials and appear to be well tolerated. (Chap. 36)

22–25. Answers

22-A; 23-B; 24-C; 25-D.

Olanzapine had the lowest QT prolongation. (Chap. 36)

26. Answer: B

Fetal exposure to valproate increases the risk of neural tube defects. (Chap. 22)

27. Answer: D

The half-life of lamotrigine increases to 66 hours when used with valproate. In comparison, the half-life of lamotrigine alone in adults is 25 to 33 hours. (Chap. 22)

28. Answer: D

The superior temporal sulcus is highly interconnected with the amygdala and the fusiform gyrus. The amygdala contributes to the recognition of others' emotional states through the analysis of facial expressions, and the lateral fusiform gyrus has a very selective role in the visual processing of faces. (Chap. 14)

29. Answer: A

Gabapentin is FDA-approved for post-herpetic neuralgia. Its use in pediatric neuropathic pain is based on case reports or case series. Tricyclic antidepressants may also be used for neuropathic pain. (Chap. 43)

30. Answer: E

A child's birth order can be relevant for a number of reasons but is the least likely to affect treatment recommendations among the options. (Chap. 27)

31. Answer: D

Although combining a stimulant with an SGA would seem to mitigate the effects of weight gain induced by an SGA, this does not appear to be the case. (Chap. 23)

32. Answer: B

Imipramine addresses both central and peripheral aspects of bladder function. (Chap. 48)

33. Answer: B

Phenelzine appears to be the most sedating of the MAOIs while tranylcypromine is the most activating. (Chap. 21)

34. Answer: A

Schizophrenia affects 1% of the population and ranks among the top 10 causes of disability worldwide. (Chap. 13)

35. Answer: C

$5-HT_{2a}$ agonists such as lysergic acid diethylamide (LSD) have hallucinogenic properties, whereas antagonist agents such as clozapine antagonize $5-HT_{2a}$, leading to interest in this receptor. Associations between clozapine response and two HTR_{2A} polymorphisms have been replicated, although they appear to make only a modest contribution to determining clozapine response. Thus, clinical utility remains elusive. (Chap. 6)

36. Answer: C

Methadone should be considered for pregnant, opiate-addicted teenagers. (Chap. 41)

37. Answer: D

Additional symptoms may include feeding difficulties and hyper- or hypotonia. (Chap. 44)

38. Answer: D

There is a strong association between the risk of developing Stevens-Johnson syndrome or toxic epidermal necrolysis and the presence of an inherited variant of the HLA-B gene (HLA-B*1502), which is largely absent in individuals not of Asian origin. Testing for HLA-B*1502 is required according to the FDA for patients of Chinese ancestry prior to initiating carbamazepine. (Chap. 22)

39. Answer: B

Histamines block the histaminergic receptors. (Chap. 24)

40. Answer: B

Bipolar II disorder requires a major depressive episode and a hypomanic episode. (Chap. 33)

41. Answer: B

Dementia praecox is not synonymous with CDI. (Chap. 38)

42. Answer: C

The NNT is the number of patients who need to be treated in order to get one response that is attributable to active treatment (and not just to the placebo effect). The NNT for fluoxetine alone is 6. (Chap. 32)

43. Answer: D

Cyproheptadine has shown utility in reducing traumatic nightmares in a small number of studies. (Chap. 39)

44. Answer: A and B

HAM-A and PARS are used to assess symptom severity in non-OCD anxiety. Answers C and D are self report. (Chap. 34)

45. Answer: C

About 30% of the glutamate contained in the brain functions as the major excitatory neurotransmitter. (Chap. 2)

46. Answer: D

Interneurons use GABA as a neurotransmitter. (Chap. 2)

47. Answer: D

Lorazepam does not increase lithium levels; however, NSAIDs, fluoxetine, ampicillin, and lisinopril do increase lithium levels. Tetracyclines, calcium channel blockers, antipsychotic agents, and propranolol, among others, also increase lithium levels. (Chap. 22)

48. Answer: C

ECT appears to be highly effective for adults with major depression. (Chap. 26)

49. Answer: D

Carbamazepine decreases lamotrigine plasma levels by 50%. (Chap. 22)

50. Answer: A

Many tics can be suppressed for brief periods of time. (Chap. 12)

51. Answer: C

Trauma exposure occurs in two-thirds of all children and 13% of these will develop some post-traumatic symptoms. (Chap. 39)

52. Answer: B

Marijuana use may precipitate latent schizophrenia in youths with EOSS. (Chap. 37)

53. Answer: D

Even children with remitted anxiety disorders remain vulnerable for later-life recurrences. (Chap. 10)

54. Answer: E

Mercury may be a contaminant in fish oil capsules. Buying from a reputable manufacturer is important, one that certifies its capsules. (Chap. 25)

55. Answer: D

The amnestic effects of ECT are greater for knowledge about the world, for recent events prior to ECT, and for less salient events. (Chap. 26)

56. Answer: E

Elevated blood alcohol levels suppress REM and slow-wave sleep but this phenomenon shifts with a decrease in blood alcohol levels. (Chap. 46)

57. Answer: C

About two-thirds of patients respond to a first stimulant. (Chap. 18)

58. Answer: A

Histone acetylation leads to the uncoiling of chromatin at a particular gene site, allowing DNA to be transcribed; it is a well-studied epigenetic mechanism. (Chap. 8)

59. Answer: C

Secretin was once touted as a treatment for autism, but evidence shows no benefit. (Chap. 25)

60. Answer: D

Osteopenia is also an emerging concern for long-term prolactin elevation. (Chap. 37)

61. Answer: D

Aside from symptom rating scales, assessments such as direct observation, time to events, counting of discrete events, and global ratings can be used to measure response to treatment. (Chap. 50)

62. Answer: C

Methylphenidate blocks the dopamine transporter and norepinephrine reuptake. (Chap. 18)

63. Answer: A

SSRIs suppress the duration of REM sleep and often prolong the onset of REM, and they may increase the number of rapid eye movements. Consequently, the increased REM density has been called "Prozac eyes." SSRIs also suppress slow-wave sleep, but this is not the reason for the latter nickname. (Chap. 46)

64. Answer: D

It has remained relatively stable since 1991 at around 75% (rates went up dramatically, especially from 1989 to 1991). Prescriptions patterns are highly variable across states, counties, and cities. (Chap. 49)

65. Answer: B

In general, choosing the medication with the shortest possible half-life can help address the "morning hangover" effect. (Chap. 46)

66. Answer: D

Stress may have a particular impact on the developing brain, which can contribute to the development of a substance abuse disorder. (Chap. 17)

67. Answer: C

Potential side effects of lithium treatment, which include weight gain and acne, can affect adherence to treatment, especially in adolescents. (Chap. 22)

68. Answer: D

The half-life of guanfacine immediate-release ranges from 10 to 30 hours in adults and from 13 to 14 hours in children. (Chap. 19)

69. Answer: C

Patients usually develop dependence within the first 3 to 4 months of chronic benzodiazepine use. (Chap. 24)

70. Answer: B

Baclofen is an agonist at the GABA$_B$ receptor. Benzodiazepines bind the GABA$_A$ receptor. (Chap. 2)

71. Answer: B

The age range of onset for childhood OCD is 7 to 12 years with a mean of 10 years; the mean age of assessment is 13 years, meaning there is a delay to assessment. The age of onset for adults averages 21 years, suggesting a bimodal distribution. (Chap. 35)

72. Answer: E

Paroxetine does not have FDA approval for disorders in children and adolescents. In adults paroxetine is approved for MDD, OCD, panic disorder, social anxiety disorder, GAD, PTSD, and premenstrual dysphoric disorder. (Chap. 20)

73. Answer: B

Physostigmine is a reversible inhibitor, while organophosphorous compounds are irreversible. (Chap. 2)

74. Answer: C

Case reports had suggested methylphenidate lowers the seizure threshold but no controlled studies have found this. It does not appear to increase the risk of seizures in children without epilepsy or in children with epileptiform discharges on EEG. (Chap. 43)

75. Answer: D

Serum valproate levels should be measured 12 hours after the last dose. (Chap. 22

76. Answer: E

Substances contained in St. John's wort have been found to interact with a number of neurotransmitter systems implicated in depression and psychiatric illness generally, but the exact mechanism remains obscure. St. John's inhibits serotonin, norepinephrine, and dopamine, but these effects seem weak. There is also an effect on GABA and MAO. (Chap. 25)

77. Answer: B

Pregabalin has not been approved for the treatment of any mood or anxiety disorder in either children or adults. (Chap. 22)

78. Answer: B

Validity describes how well a screening or diagnostic instrument actually measures what it is intended to measure. (Chap. 28)

79. Answer: C

The answer option of 0.8 is the one that corresponds to a medium-large effect size. (Chap. 47)

80. Answer: D

In treatment-resistant patients, clozapine blood levels should typically be greater than 350 ng/dL. (Chap. 37)

81. Answer: C

Whether or not the treatment will be used by a given family cannot be answered in a clinical trial. (Chap. 50)

82. Answer: A and C

Lower IQ (<50) and lower mental age (≤4.5 years) were modestly associated with worse response to psychostimulants. (Chap. 42)

83. Answer: B

Clomipramine acts at both serotonin and norepinephrine receptors. (Chap. 35)

84. Answer: B

The approximate relative risk of suicidal thinking and behaviors on SSRIs compared to placebo is 2. (Chap. 20)

85. Answer: D

There are a number of physiological systems involved in trauma. (Chap. 39)

86. Answer: A

Children with comorbid diagnoses of dysthymic disorder and MDD, often called "double depression," have a greater risk for a protracted course. (Chap. 32)

87. Answer: D

An absolute reading of >500 msec or an increase from baseline of >60 msec should prompt discontinuation. For values between 450 and 500 msec, agents with greater QTc prolongation, such as ziprasidone or clozapine, should be avoided or carefully monitored. If values between 450 or 500 msec develop during treatment, whether to continue will depend on the unique clinical benefit of the agent and other risk factors. (Chap. 23)

88. Answer: B

The antidepressant efficacy of MAOI medications was critical in developing the monoamine hypothesis for mood disorders. Iproniazid was FDA-approved as an antidepressant in 1957. (Chap. 21)

89. Answer: A

An anticholinergic agent is given during ECT to decrease bronchial secretions and attenuate the increased vagal activity. (Chap. 26)

90–93. Answers

90-A (partial agonist); 91-B (partial agonist); 92-B (partial agonist); 93-C (agonist). (Chap. 2)

94–96. Answers

94-B and D; 95-C; 96-A. (Chap. 2)

97. Answer: B

SSRIs have not been shown to be effective for weight restoration, depression, or other symptoms in anorexia nervosa. Interestingly, one study found that patients without anorexia who are depressed and on a hypocaloric diet also do not respond to SSRIs. (Chap. 40)

98. Answer: A

Citalopram, escitalopram, paroxetine, sertraline, and venlafaxine have the least CYP450 inhibition among the answer options. (Chap. 43)

99. Answer: D

Fluoxetine inhibits CYP3A isozymes and thus increases the plasma concentration of triazolobenzodiazepines, which include alprazolam, midazolam, and triazolam. (Chap. 24)

100. Answer: D

Lamotrigine is a substrate of both UGT1A4 and UGT2B7 and levels are increased in the presence of valproic acid. (Chap. 4)

101. Answer: C

TMS was first used in the mid-1980s to assess the integrity of motor pathways in the CNS prior to its use for psychiatric illness. (Chap. 26)

102. Answer: C

A number of neurotransmitter systems have been implicated in Tourette's disorder. (Chap. 12)

103. Answer: A

Clomipramine used alone or with an SSRI would be your next step. A third SSRI is less likely to be effective. Venlafaxine and duloxetine can be considered. Like clomipramine, they have dual serotonin and norepinephrine activity but have less problematic management issues and side effects. They have the support of expert opinion but no randomized controlled trial data. Atypical agents could also be considered as an augmentation strategy to an SSRI—but not alone—if two failed trials of SSRIs have been demonstrated. (Chap. 35)

104. Answer: B

Clearance by an organ such as the liver or kidney is defined as the volume of blood that is totally "cleared" of drug per unit of time. (Chap. 3)

105. Answer: B

Fetal-placental circulation is established by 21 days' gestation and continues to develop until the fourth month of pregnancy. Obviously this has relevance to psychopharmacological decision-making for the pregnant patient. (Chap. 44)

106. Answer: C

Starvation induces mood symptoms, especially depression, often followed by isolation and withdrawal. (Chap. 40)

107. Answer: B

The Course of Bipolar Illness in Youth (COBY) study found that >50% of youths with bipolar I disorder had a prior history of a major depressive episode. (Chap. 33)

108. Answer: D

*In a SMART trial subjects are randomized to an intervention and are later randomized to a second intervention or control condition depending on their response to the first treatment. STAR*D is an example of a SMART design, as is TEAM (Treatment of Early Age Mania). (Chap. 50)*

109. Answer: B

After 5 years of age, the total brain volume changes minimally, but the two dynamic processes persisting into young adulthood are synaptic pruning and myelination. (Chap. 9)

110–113. Answers

110-C; 111-D; 112-B; 113-A. (*Chap. 28*)

114. Answer: B

According to the American Medical Association (AMA) CME activities consist of educational activities that serve to maintain, develop, or increase the knowledge, skills, and professional performance and relationships a physician uses to provide services for patients, the public, or the profession. (Chap. 53)

115. Answer: A

The majority of suicidal adverse events when taking SSRIs were increases in ideation; less common were attempts, and there were no completed suicides. (Chap. 32)

116. Answer: D

Benzodiazepines and anticonvulsant medications inhibit seizure induction and can shorten seizure duration, resulting in decreased treatment effectiveness of ECT. (Chap. 26)

117. Answer: B

The high-potency first-generation antipsychotics such as haloperidol and fluphenazine appear to have the greatest risk for EPS. (Chap. 37)

118. Answer: D

Continuous or dimensional measures are rating scales such as weight or blood pressure. (Chap. 28)

119. Answer: C

Liver injury on atomoxetine has been reported in at least two cases (of 3 million patients). Both patients recovered after atomoxetine was stopped, but the potential for liver failure is present. The manufacturer added a warning about this possibility. Part of prescribing may include discussing with families the signs to look for, including yellowing of skin and sclera. (Chap. 31)

120. Answer: D

This prevalence greatly exceeds the rate found in the general population; however, the reliability of making such a diagnosis in people with intellectual disability is confounded by the presence of behaviors confused with the negative symptoms of schizophrenia. (Chap. 42)

121. Answer: D

The three subtypes of specific phobia are animal, blood/ injection/injury, and environmental/situational phobias. (Chap. 10)

122. Answer: C

OCD is a brain disorder involving the frontal-subcortical circuits. (Chap. 11)

123. Answer: D

A prospective case series (Spiller et al., 2005) of clonidine ingestion reported to poison control centers highlights its potential for serious adverse effects in children, including coma, even at doses as low as 0.3 mg. This is one reason to titrate clonidine; however, higher doses have been used clinically and may be indicated for a given patient. (Chap. 45)

124. Answer: B

Stimulants should be prescribed judiciously, after consideration, in patients with known heart defects. (Chap. 31)

125. Answer: E

Carbamazepine is one of the traditional agents, which include lithium and valproate. The novel agents also include gabapentin. (Chap. 22)

126. Answer: D

Providing eight Internet interactive online sessions to patients with bulimia, with peer and parent support through message boards, has been shown to be effective. The other approaches have not been evaluated. (Chap. 40)

127. Answer: A

All the other scales are widely available to evaluate the neuromotor side effects of antipsychotics. (Chap. 23)

128. Answer: B

The National Center for Complementary and Alternative Medicine (NCCAM) was established in 1998. (Chap. 25)

129. Answer: C

P-glycoprotein acts as a gatekeeper to a drug's contact with intestinal CYP enzymes. (Chap. 4)

130. Answer: B

The range of placebo response in pediatric OCD has been reported to be 25% to 37%. (Chap. 35)

131. Answer: A

Onset of drinking by age 14 signifies a poor prognosis. The other answer options are phrased oppositely to what is accurate. (Chap. 41)

132. Answer: B

The adverse event profiles of antipsychotics limit their usefulness in ADHD; however, they are used in refractory cases and where other symptoms are present, such as comorbid bipolar disorder, severe mood dysregulation, and aggression. Studies have shown that they are effective in certain subpopulations of children with ADHD. (Chap. 31)

133. Answer: C

Benzodiazepines are mostly absorbed in the GI tract. Lorazepam is also available in a sublingual form that reaches clinical effect at the same rate as an oral dose. (Chap. 2)

134. Answer: C

The term that describes the probability that a child identified by a screening instrument as having a disorder actually has the disorder is called the positive predictive power. (Chap. 28)

135. Answer: E

The best example, as described in the textbook, is the development of the ocular dominance columns within the visual cortical system during the critical period. (Chap. 1)

136. Answer: D

The Course of Bipolar Illness in Youth (COBY) study found that youths with bipolar disorder spent more time symptomatic and had greater mixed or cycling episodes than adults with bipolar disorder. (Chap. 33)

137. Answer: C

In structural imaging, global reduction in total brain volume, affecting gray and white matter equally, has been found in subjects with ADHD. (Chap. 11)

138. Answer: E

Alpha agonists have not been used as a part of standard practice in major depressive disorder. Alpha agonists do not have FDA approval for use in PTSD, ODD, and conduct disorder and are used off-label for these disorders. (Chap. 19)

139. Answer: B

Atypical antipsychotic augmentation should be used judiciously in children. Clinical experience indicates that a minimum of two different adequate SSRI trials or an SSRI and clomipramine should be used before atypical augmentation. (Chap. 35)

140. Answer: A

Interactions between gene and environment resulting in changes in gene expression apart from changes in DNA are termed epigenetic. (Chap. 15)

141. Answer: A

Phase 0 trials are relatively new and are meant to speed the development of drugs that prove promising in preclinical studies; about 10 subjects are usually enrolled. They are not meant to offer data on therapeutic efficacy but provide information about pharmacokinetic action in humans. (Chap. 50)

142. Answer: C

Pharmacodynamic studies focus on genetic variations at the sites of drug action. Most studies examine neuronal receptors and transporters. (Chap. 6)

143. Answer: A

Although the distinction between atypical and typical is blurred in some respects, clozapine is considered the first atypical antipsychotic.

144. Answer: D

A switch to another SSRI is indicated when a child with OCD does not respond to one SSRI. (Chap. 35)

145. Answer: C

However, the increase in panic attacks around puberty infrequently progress to panic disorder. (Chap. 10)

146. Answer: B

Young children are sensitive to contextual factors such as time of day (due to nap and feeding schedules) or being in new settings, so multiple visits will contribute toward a more accurate assessment. (Chap. 45)

147. Answer: A

There has been an increase in the prescription rate for preschoolers across drug classes. Stimulants account for much of this increase, but antipsychotics and other agents have shown an increase as well. (Chap. 49)

148. Answer: B

Prolongations of the PR interval and the QTc have been reported in some individuals, but consistent effects have not been observed in systematic studies. (Chap. 19)

149. Answer: C

Options A and B describe the approach of pragmatic and ideal clinical trials. (Chap. 29)

150. Answer: A and C

Body fat and total body water affect drug distribution; gastric emptying time and drug polarity affect the rate of absorption of the drug. (Chap. 3)

151. Answer: D

Clonidine is generally tapered unless used only briefly, less than a week. (Chap. 19)

152. Answer: A

Although midazolam is not the first choice among benzodiazepines, it is an option. Droperidol was used regularly for emergencies in adults but fell out of favor due to its effects on cardiac conduction. (Chap. 47)

153. Answer: D

An industry-sponsored controlled trial as well as an open trial of ziprasidone failed to demonstrate efficacy in children with EOSS. (Chap. 37)

154. Answer: B

The non-benzodiazepine hypnotics have little effect on sleep architecture. Other advantages are that tolerance does not develop for at least a month and there is no withdrawal syndrome when they are discontinued. (Chap. 2)

155. Answer: B

The effect size for sertraline in one large double-blind study of youth was 0.45. (Chap. 24)

156. Answer: D

Trimipramine also does not have established therapeutic blood levels. A steady-state level for tricyclic antidepressants is normally reached after 5 days' administration, at which time a level can be checked when applicable. (Chap. 21)

157. Answer: B

Ramelteon binds to melatonin 1 and 2 receptors. The binding at the melatonin 1 site by ramelteon is approximately six times as strong as the binding of melatonin to this site. (Chap. 2)

158. Answer: A

Pharmacokinetics can be defined as what the body does to the drug. (Chap. 3)

159. Answer: C

Separation anxiety disorder and selective mutism are anxiety disorders and are defined under "Disorders Usually First Diagnosed in Infancy and Childhood." (Chap. 34)

160. Answer: C

Anxiety may lead to reduced oxygenation. (Chap. 43)

161. Answer: E

Either an atypical antipsychotic or a mood stabilizer is recommended by CABF. (Chap. 33)

162. Answer: A

Intermittent explosive disorder (or episodic dyscontrol syndrome) is aggression that results in serious assaults or property destruction in the face of limited provocation and that is usually accompanied by remorse. (Chap. 47)

163. Answer: B

There are five risk categories reflecting the degree of risk to the fetus based on animal and human data: A, B, C, D, and X. However these guidelines are being reviewed because experts believe this rating system can be misleading because it does not elucidate the differences between the risk categories. (Chap. 44)

164. Answer: A

Escitalopram has FDA approval for major depressive disorder in children 12 to 17 years of age. It is approved for GAD and MDD in adults. (Chap. 20)

165. Answer: B

Plasma steady-state concentration describes the equilibrium between the amount of drug ingested and the amount of drug eliminated. (Chap. 3)

166. Answer: B

Intravenous administration produces the equivalent of 100% absorption. (Chap. 3)

167. Answer: A

Longitudinally, symptoms of ADHD may improve but substance use remains the same. (Chap. 41)

168. Answer: C

An important clinical component discussed in Chapter 30 is the power of the placebo effect even when patients know they are taking placebo. (Chap. 30)

169. Answer: D

A significant proportion of child psychiatric inpatients are victims of abuse, more than half of patients. (Chap. 8)

170. Answer: D

The effectiveness of monoamine oxidase inhibitors for depression was discovered in the 1960s. (Chap. 21)

171. Answer: B

Mutations in MC4R gene occur in approximately 1% of obese adults and in 2% to 6% of obese children. (Chap. 16)

172. Answer: A

The use of naltrexone for self-injurious behaviors is based on the notion that this class of patients has an elevated threshold for pain or that self-injury produces surges of endorphins that reinforce the behavior. (Chap. 42)

173. Answer: B

Options A and C are efficacious in preventing depressive relapse. (Chap. 32)

174. Answer: D

Over 70% of 17-month-old children in this sample were physically aggressive to peers, siblings, and adults. (Chap. 15)

175. Answer: D

MAOIs can cause a hypertensive crisis when combined with the above-mentioned tyramine-containing foods (as well as wines and some legumes) and also with monoamine agonists such as stimulants. (Chap. 21)

176. Answer: C

Tic elimination is not a reasonable expectation of treatment because elimination is unlikely. Medications are not used for prophylaxis. (Chap. 36)

177. Answer: A

Synergism is not a biochemical inhibition mechanism. (Chap. 4)

178. Answer: D

Moreover, antipsychotic medications and occasionally SSRIs can also cause constipation. (Chap. 48)

179. Answer: B

Inattention, hyperactivity, and impulsiveness, which are defining features of ADHD, would also be a focus of stimulant treatment. The tantrums, aggression, and self-injury in autism, which are often target problems of medication treatment, are NOT defining features of autism; a similar logic applies to the other options. (Chap. 27)

180. Answer: A

NNT represents the number of patients who need to be treated by an intervention to produce one additional favorable outcome beyond that of the control condition. (Chap. 29)

181. Answer: C

Melatonin binds to receptors in the suprachiasmatic nucleus in the hypothalamus. (Chap. 46)

182. Answer: E

Levonorgestrel is a substrate of CYP3A4, which topiramate induces. Induction takes several days to take effect and takes time to resolve, since it involves the induction of proteins. (Chap. 4)

183. Answer: C

The Child Behavior Checklist covers a wide range of behavior problems and is not a mania-specific screening instrument. (Chap. 33)

184. Answer: C

The prefrontal cortex regulates attention and executive functioning. (Chap. 11)

185. Answer: D

The data suggest that there are pockets of over-prescription, but equally concerning from a public health perspective is that many children who need treatment are not receiving it. (Chap. 49)

186. Answer: C

In the MTA, behavioral interventions were helpful for children with comorbid conditions but not so much for core symptoms of ADHD. Modafinil was not used in the MTA. (Chap. 18)

187. Answer: A

Duloxetine is an SNRI. (Chap. 21)

188. Answer: C

Ziprasidone does not appear to be effective in adolescents. (Chap. 37)

189. Answer: C

Interestingly, exposure to either an SSRI or a benzodiazepine <u>separately</u> was not associated with either congenital anomalies as a group or a cardiac defect specifically. (Chap. 44)

190. Answer: D

Phase II metabolism involves conjugation with endogenous substrates such as sulfate, acetate, or glucuronic acid. (Chap. 3)

191. Answer: B

Bupropion should not be administered with an MAOI as both have noradrenergic and dopaminergic action, which may increase the risk of a hypertensive crisis. (Chap. 21)

192. Answer: C

The familial risk of schizophrenia spectrum disorders is greater for probands with childhood-onset than adult-onset schizophrenia. (Chap. 13)

193. Answer: D

Zaleplon (Sonata) is a non-benzodiazepine receptor agonist with a short half-life, and eszopiclone (Lunesta) is a non-benzodiazepine receptor agonist with a longer half-life approved for sleep maintenance as well as sleep initiation insomnia. (Chap. 46)

194. Answer: A

Patients assigned to placebo will be receiving an inferior treatment. Families may refuse enrollment knowing other treatment exists, thus reducing the representativeness of the sample. (For depression studies in adolescents, placebo leads to a high response rate and is considered acceptable for this reason.) (Chap. 50)

195. Answer: A

Sertraline or CBT was superior to placebo, but the combination performed best. (Chap. 34)

196. Answer: D

The definition of dysfunctional voiding consists of those three statements. (Chap. 48)

197. Answer: B

Trimipramine is a tertiary amine. (Chap. 21)

198. Answer: B

Disulfiram prevents the breakdown of acetaldehyde, a toxic metabolite, and leads to a number of unpleasant effects that make drinking alcohol aversive. Ethanol is metabolized to acetaldehyde by alcohol dehydrogenase; acetaldehyde is metabolized to acetic acid by aldehyde dehydrogenase. One small randomized trial, with positive results, has been conducted in youths. Its potential lethality makes its use likely limited to inpatient settings or intensive outpatient treatment with a closely involved family. (Chap. 41)

199. Answer: D

The cognitive effects of alpha agonists are mostly mediated by post-synaptic alpha-2a receptors. (Chap. 19)

200. Answer: B

Hyperphagia is not a phenomenon of dopamine rebound. (Chap. 23)

Test 6 Questions

1. What is the mechanism of action of gabapentin?

   A. Modulates norepinephrine influx and influences GABA-ergic transmission

   B. Modulates calcium influx and influences GABA-ergic transmission

   C. Modulates serotonin reuptake

   D. Modulates dopamine and GABA-ergic transmission

2. Youths with maladaptive aggression present a greater annual cost to society than do youths without conduct disturbance. What is the approximate ratio of this cost?

   A. 2:1

   B. 6:1

   C. 60:1

   D. 600:1

3. Which of the following options best characterizes the American Academy of Child and Adolescent Psychiatry's (AACAP) Practice Parameters for initiation of a stimulant?

   A. Baseline assessment of current symptoms, appetite, sleep, height, weight, and cardiovascular status history

   B. Baseline assessment of current symptoms and cardiovascular status history

   C. Baseline assessment of current symptoms, height, weight, and cardiovascular status history

   D. Baseline assessment of current symptoms of ADHD, appetite, sleep, height, and weight

4. There has been an increase in the prescription of psychotropics for children. To determine whether this represents good or bad clinical practice requires all the following EXCEPT:

   A. Determine the extent of psychiatric disorders

   B. Determine whether children without a *bona fide* psychiatric disorder are being treated

   C. Determine the physician or practitioner specialty doing the prescribing

   D. Determine which treatments work for which condition, based on controlled trials

   E. Determine which treatment is considered the treatment of choice

5. Which of the following statements best describes the concept of internal validity in clinical research?

   A. The effectiveness of an intervention under usual conditions

   B. The effectiveness of an intervention under ideal conditions

   C. The extent to which results can be generalized to clinical populations

   D. The extent to which a study is methodologically sound

6. All the following are psychosocial interventions that have an evidence base for the treatment of aggressive youth EXCEPT:

   A. Cognitive problem-solving skills

   B. Functional family therapy

   C. Group therapy

   D. Anger management

   E. Multisystemic therapy

7. Which of the following most closely describes treatment as usual (TAU) in clinical trials?

   A. Treatment that is considered the standard of care and delivered in the community

   B. Assessment and referral to whatever treatment the family can find in the community

   C. Treatment delivered by study personnel according to established standards of care

   D. Continuing the treatment the family was receiving before enrollment

8. In the "classic" view of basal ganglia function there are two pathways that link striatal output to the thalamus. The direct is GABA-ergic and inhibitory. Neurons in the direct pathway are conceptualized as bearing D1 receptors and co-expressing substance P and dynorphin. The indirect pathway is excitatory through glutamate. Neurons are conceptualized as having D2 receptors and co-expressing enkephalin. This model has been modified in which manner?

   A. D1 and D2 are found together in both pathways.

   B. Rather than directly inhibiting striatal neurons, dopamine is now viewed as modulating the interaction of glutamate and dopamine receptors and the function of GABA and serotonin neurons.

   C. Other interneurons, such as cholinergic ones, have been identified.

   D. Nitrous oxide inhibits the uptake of dopamine, norepinephrine, and serotonin and is closely linked to glutamate transmission.

   E. All of the above

9. Exposure to most drugs of abuse leads to activation of dopaminergic cells in which part of the brain?

   A. Prefrontal cortex

   B. Ventral tegmental area

   C. Amygdala

   D. Locus coeruleus

10. There have been longstanding concerns about stimulant-associated growth deficits in children with ADHD. Which of the following best characterizes the knowledge base about the issue?

    A. Stimulants have been found to affect circadian rhythms of growth-hormone release.

    B. Stimulants have been found to affect nutrient absorption.

    C. No consistent neurohormonal pathophysiology has been identified to explain stimulant-associated height deficits.

    D. Stimulants increase decrease cyclic adenosine monophosphate activity.

11. Which of the following is first-line treatment for pediatric nocturnal enuresis?

    A. Imipramine

    B. Bell-and-pad device

    C. Restriction of fluids 3 hours before bedtime

    D. Atropine

12. Gabapentin is structurally similar to:

    A. Glutamate

    B. Imipramine

    C. Monoamine oxidase inhibitors

    D. Carbamazepine

    E. GABA

13. Specific phobias in children generally cluster into three subtypes. Which one can result in physiological symptomatology including initial rise in heart rate, followed by vasovagal bradycardia, and syncope?

    A. Animal phobias

    B. Blood/injection/injury phobias

    C. Environmental/situational phobias

14. The half-life of lamotrigine in adults is 25 to 33 hours. What is the half-life in children aged 5 to 11 years?

    A. 25 to 33 hours

    B. 18 to 23 hours

    C. 14 hours

    D. 7 hours

    E. 3 to 6 hours

15. Which antipsychotic is likely to have the greatest risk for extrapyramidal symptoms?

    A. Olanzapine

    B. Quetiapine

    C. Ziprasidone

    D. Aripiprazole

16. Which of the following best captures the state of empiric support for pediatric psychopharmacology in posttraumatic stress disorder (PTSD)? From 1980 to 2009 there have been:

    A. <20 articles on medication treatment of PTSD

    B. 100 to 500 articles on medication treatment

    C. 500 to 1000 articles on medication treatment

    D. 1000 or more articles on medication treatment

17. Methylphenidate, D-methylphenidate, and D-amphetamine are short-acting compounds with which of the following profiles of action?

    A. Onset of action within 30 to 60 minutes, peak clinical effect after 1 to 2 hours, lasting 2 to 5 hours

    B. Onset of action within 30 to 60 minutes, peak clinical effect after 3 to 5 hours, lasting 6 to 8 hours

    C. Onset of action within 5 to 15 minutes, peak clinical effect after 30 minutes to 1 hour, lasting 3 to 5 hours

    D. Onset of action within 1 to 2 hours, peak clinical effect after 2 to 4 hours, lasting 8 to 10 hours

18. Which of the following is the only Schedule IV approved hypnotic to promote sleep?

    A. Zolpidem

    B. Lorazepam

    C. Eszopiclone

    D. Ramelteon

19. The American Academy of Child and Adolescent Psychiatry established which group to address the increasing use of psychotropic medications in a subpopulation of children?

    A. Elementary School Psychopharmacology Working Group

    B. Preschool Psychopharmacology Working Group

    C. High School Psychopharmacology Working Group

    D. College Student Psychopharmacology Working Group

20. Which of the following medications is considered a traditional mood stabilizer?

    A. Lamotrigine

    B. Oxcarbazepine

    C. Valproate

    D. Pregabalin

    E. Topiramate

21. The idea that certain actions are always morally right or wrong independent of outcomes is related to:

    A. Common sense

    B. Deontology

    C. Utilitarianism

    D. Justice

22. Which of the following has been shown to protect against drug-seeking behaviors in mice?

    A. Enriched environment early in life

    B. Separation from mothers early in life

    C. Introduction of psychostimulants early in life

    D. A and C

23. After the first year of monitoring absolute neutrophil counts (ANC) in patients on clozapine treatment, how often should ANC be monitored?

    A. Weekly

    B. Every 2 weeks

    C. Every 4 weeks

    D. No monitoring needed after the first year of normal results

24. Phase I metabolic reactions are best defined as:

    A. Initial absorption of a drug

    B. The disruption of a monovalent bond to expose an oxygen group for further phase II processing

    C. Breaking off a part of a drug and uncovering or inserting a chemical structure that acts as a functional handle for further phase II processing

    D. The addition of a divalent bond to expose an oxygen group for further phase II processing

25. All of the following are metabolic adverse effects in antipsychotic treatment EXCEPT:

    A. Hypoglycemia

    B. Metabolic syndrome

    C. Diabetes

    D. Dyslipidemia

26. Dopamine is formed from which amino acid?

    A. Lysine

    B. Tryptophan

    C. Tyrosine

    D. Glutamate

27. A psychiatrist has a patient with major depression who smokes one pack of cigarettes a day. Given this limited information, which of the following options might be considered as a first choice?

    A. Mirtazapine

    B. Lithium

    C. Duloxetine

    D. Bupropion

28. Norepinephrine is produced from:

    A. Serotonin

    B. Dopamine

    C. Epinephrine

    D. Acetylcholine

29. The prevalence of stimulant prescriptions is greatest in the United States compared to other industrialized countries. What is one explanation?

    A. Stimulants are cheaper in the United States.

    B. More extensive health coverage in United States

    C. More equitable income distribution in the United States

    D. Diagnostic differences between DSM and ICD

30. A recent study of self-reports of physical violence during early childhood to early adulthood found which TWO factors were inversely associated with a high frequency of physical violence?

    A. Executive functioning

    B. Nonverbal IQ

    C. Verbal IQ

    D. Visual-motor integration

31. The co-administration of guanfacine and valproic acid may lead to which of the following?

    A. Increase in valproic acid

    B. Decrease in valproic acid

    C. Increase in guanfacine

    D. Decrease in guanfacine

32. Ethinyl estradiol in oral contraceptives (OCs) can induce glucuronidation and lower the plasma levels of which drug?

    A. Topiramate

    B. Fluoxetine

    C. Sertraline

    D. Lamotrigine

    E. Alprazolam

33. In which of the following antidepressants is discontinuation syndrome most common upon abrupt cessation?

    A. Mirtazapine

    B. Bupropion

    C. Venlafaxine

    D. Duloxetine

34. All of these are symptom clusters of posttraumatic stress disorder (PTSD) in children EXCEPT:

    A. Avoidance and numbing

    B. Hyperarousal

    C. Re-experiencing

    D. Somatic

35. In a clinical trial, what is a type I error?

    A. Rejecting the null hypothesis when the difference is in fact due to chance

    B. Failing to reject the null hypothesis when there is a real difference between treatment groups

    C. The ability to detect a difference due to chance

    D. The ability to detect a difference due to real effect

36. 22q11 deletion syndrome or velo-cardio-facial syndrome occurs in 1 in 4000 births and is a known risk factor for which of the following?

    A. Schizophrenia

    B. Autism

    C. Intellectual disability

    D. All of the above

37. Regarding stimulant use for attention-deficit/hyperactivity disorder (ADHD) when a comorbid seizure disorder is present, which of the following statements are TRUE?

    A. Package inserts contraindicate the use of stimulants.

    B. Stimulants may be safe in children with a known seizure disorder whose seizures are well controlled.

    C. When epilepsy is uncontrolled, stimulants may worsen seizures.

    D. All of the above

38. Before human subjects are enrolled in an investigation, institutional review boards (IRBs) assess risks to the subjects, potential benefits to subjects and society, the knowledge that may be gained from the research, and the adequacy of the informed consent process to be used. After initial approval, studies must undergo continuing reviews by IRBs how often?

    A. Every 3 months

    B. Every 6 months

    C. Annually

    D. Every 2 years

39. Which of the following statements about benzodiazepine use in the treatment of initial insomnia is accurate?

    A. Tolerance to the sleep improvements may occur in 1 to 3 weeks.

    B. There is a decrease in the amount of stage 2 sleep.

    C. There is excessive daytime alertness.

    D. There is an increase of sleep efficiency.

40. Which of the following is a recommended practice for discontinuing tricyclic antidepressants in patients?

    A. Prompt discontinuation over 1 to 2 days

    B. Decreasing the dose by 10 to 25 mg every 2 to 3 days

    C. Cross-tapering with fluoxetine

    D. Slow discontinuation over 3 to 6 months

41. Which two agents have the least QTc prolongation?

    A. Risperidone and thioridazine

    B. Quetiapine and risperidone

    C. Olanzapine and oral aripiprazole

    D. Chlorpromazine and olanzapine

For the following questions match the drug with the correct FDA labeling for children and/or adolescents. A drug may have more than one correct corresponding answer option, or an answer option may correspond to more than one drug. (Note: The approved age ranges are not specified in the answer options for simplicity.)

42. Fluoxetine

43. Escitalopram

44. Atomoxetine

45. Divalproex sodium

46. Fluvoxamine

    A. Efficacy was not established for pediatric bipolar disorder.

    B. Approved for obsessive-compulsive disorder

    C. Approved for major depressive disorder

    D. Approved for attention-deficit/hyperactivity disorder

47. **All the following are side effects of benzodiazepine withdrawal EXCEPT:**

    A. Insomnia

    B. Trembling

    C. Dry skin

    D. Dry mouth

    E. Palpitations

48. **A cohort study of pregnant women found that maternal benzodiazepine use during pregnancy was associated with:**

    A. Increased risk of preterm delivery

    B. Low Apgar scores

    C. Increased risk of low birth weight

    D. All of the above

49. **Which population of children is more prone to develop neurological adverse effects during the initiation phase of lithium treatment?**

    A. Preschool children

    B. Latency-age children

    C. Early adolescents

    D. Late adolescents

50. **True or False. Routine monitoring of prolactin levels is recommended for older children prescribed risperidone.**

    A. True

    B. False

51. **Which of the following selective serotonin reuptake inhibitor (SSRI) medications demonstrated the lowest ratio of umbilical cord to maternal serum concentration in a small study of pregnant women?**

    A. Sertraline

    B. Fluoxetine

    C. Citalopram

    D. Paroxetine

52. **Which of the following statements about alpha-2 adrenergic receptors is FALSE?**

    A. There are three receptor subtypes of alpha-2.

    B. They are composed of seven transmembrane domains.

    C. Polypeptide chains are coupled to G proteins.

    D. Antagonist binding to a receptor terminal leads to the exchange of guanine diphosphate for guanine triphosphate on the alpha subunit.

53. **Motivational interviewing has a growing evidence base in pediatric behavioral health for enhancing medication adherence, using all the following therapeutic components EXCEPT:**

    A. Empathy that matches the patient's experience

    B. Positive expectations regarding the recommended treatment

    C. Patient confidence in his or her ability to improve

    D. Insight upon the latent conflicts that obstruct symptom improvement

54. **Which CYP enzyme involved in antipsychotic clearance appears to be most affected by genetic polymorphisms?**

    A. 3A4

    B. 1A2

    C. 2D6

    D. 3A5

    E. 1A1

55. **What are the optimal serum levels of valproate in order to treat mania in adults?**

    A. 65 to 85 mg/mL

    B. 75 to 95 mg/mL

    C. 80 to 100 mg/mL

    D. 85 to 110 mg/mL

    E. 100 to 115 mg/mL

56. **The alpha-2 adrenergic agonist guanfacine, in comparison with clonidine, has:**

    A. A shorter half-life

    B. A longer half-life

    C. An equivalent half-life

    D. None of the above

57. Six-month-old infants of prenatally depressed mothers demonstrate which of the following symptoms compared with infants of non-depressed mothers?

    A. Greater negative affect

    B. Heightened cortisol response to novel stimuli

    C. Reduced behavioral response to pain

    D. A and B

58. What is the most common side effect of clonidine?

    A. Hypotension

    B. Dry mouth

    C. Confusion

    D. Sedation

59. Based on the dopamine hypothesis of psychosis, the goal to reduce overactive dopamine transmission upon antipsychotic initiation is intended for which area of the brain?

    A. Mesocortical

    B. Mesolimbic

    C. Tuberoinfundibular

    D. Nigrostriatal

60. Anorexia is categorized into two subgroups, one of which is:

    A. Bulimic type

    B. Binge/purging type

    C. Restricting/bulimic type

    D. Bulimic/purging type

61. Crime statistics in the United States show what percentage of victims of sexual assault are persons under the age of 18?

    A. 15%

    B. 33%

    C. 67%

    D. 93%

62. Generally, when stimulants are effective for aggression the effect correlates to:

    A. The severity of the ADHD

    B. The presence of comorbid conduct disorder

    C. The use of a long-acting formulation

    D. There is no correlation

63. Among children and adolescents who are prescribed psychotropic medications, what percentage receive two or more agents?

    A. <5%

    B. 10% to 20%

    C. 35% to 50%

    D. >50%

64. The elimination of all of the following drugs is determined by zero-order or non-linear kinetics EXCEPT:

    A. Phenytoin

    B. Salicylate

    C. Ethanol

    D. Lithium

65. Which of the following is commonly used for tics in Europe but is not available in the United States?

    A. Sulpiride

    B. Ziprasidone

    C. Aripiprazole

    D. Fluphenazine

66. Which of the following is the most serious potential side effect of transcranial magnetic stimulation (TMS)?

    A. Headache

    B. Scalp pain

    C. Seizure

    D. Stroke

67. Most studies investigating the benefit of monoamine oxidase inhibitors (MAOIs) in youths have been for what indication?

    A. Major depressive disorder

    B. Attention-deficit/hyperactivity disorder

    C. Obsessive-compulsive disorder

    D. Panic disorder

68. What is the function of monoamine oxidase (MAO)?

    A. Inhibit the reuptake of biogenic amines

    B. Promote the reuptake of biogenic amines

    C. Inactivate endogenous and exogenous biogenic amines

    D. Up-regulate the serotonin transporter

69. What are reasons for the scant empiric support for the treatment of anorexia nervosa?

    A. Variable patient population

    B. Low prevalence

    C. Patient reluctance to seek help

    D. All of the above

70. Based on a systematic review of 10 studies in which 783 youths were followed for at least 11 months, what is the annualized rate of tardive dyskinesia in children and adolescents?

    A. 15%

    B. 10%

    C. 7%

    D. 0.4%

71. Which of the following brain regions create "neural programs" to carry out habitual behaviors?

    A. Inferior temporal cortex

    B. Posterior parietal association cortex

    C. Prefrontal cortex

    D. Basal ganglia

72. Which of the following classes of medications has the best evidence for effectiveness in pediatric anxiety?

    A. Tricyclic antidepressants

    B. Serotonin reuptake inhibitors

    C. Benzodiazepines

    D. Alpha agonists

73. What is the usual frequency of electroconvulsive therapy (ECT) sessions?

    A. Once weekly

    B. Two or three times weekly

    C. Five times weekly

    D. Daily

74. Alpha-2 adrenergic agonists stimulate secretion of which of the following?

    A. Growth hormone

    B. Oxytocin

    C. Vasopressin

    D. Prolactin

75. What is the point prevalence of obsessive-compulsive disorder in the pediatric population?

    A. 2%

    B. 7%

    C. 20%

    D. 33%

76. The co-administration of St. John's wort with other medications might result in all the following EXCEPT:

    A. Reduced risk of pregnancy on oral contraceptives

    B. Serotonin syndrome with antidepressants

    C. Organ rejection post-transplant

    D. Increased viral load in HIV

77. Which of the following antipsychotics has evidence of superior effectiveness in managing suicidality in adults?

    A. Olanzapine

    B. Clozapine

    C. Risperidone

    D. Quetiapine

78. What is the main reason physicians should avoid accepting gifts, entertainment, and industry-sponsored activities that are free of charge?

    A. It takes time away from clinical practice.

    B. Marketing influences decisions.

    C. Physicians have enough money to pay for items or activities.

    D. To please government regulators

79. All the following are symptom dimensions in obsessive-compulsive disorder (OCD) that are stable over time EXCEPT:

    A. Contamination/washing

    B. Aggression/checking

    C. Symmetry/ordering

    D. Sexuality

    E. Hoarding

80. Which of the following statements is most accurate based on clinical trial data of the Tourette Syndrome Study Group?

    A. Clonidine used alone for ADHD is superior to stimulant treatment.

    B. Methylphenidate used alone for ADHD is inferior to behavioral therapy.

    C. Methylphenidate used alone for ADHD is equivalent to clonidine and methylphenidate combination treatment.

    D. Combination treatment with clonidine and methylphenidate for ADHD is superior to methylphenidate or clonidine alone.

81. A bowel program to address pediatric constipation involves all of the following EXCEPT:

    A. Plenty of fluids

    B. Use of stool softeners

    C. Use of the gastrocolic reflex

    D. Rare use of laxatives

82. All the following are true about benzodiazepines EXCEPT:

    A. They are highly lipid-soluble.

    B. They cross the blood–brain barrier quickly.

    C. They are highly bound to plasma proteins.

    D. They have a decreased accumulation in obese individuals.

83. The American Medical Student Association scores academic medical centers on their conflict-of-interest policies. All of the following are viewed as creating potentially significant conflicts of interest EXCEPT:

    A. Samples

    B. Sales representatives

    C. National Institutes of Health grants

    D. Consulting relationships

    E. Industry support

84. What percentage of the entire body content of serotonin is found in the central nervous system (CNS)?

    A. 95%

    B. 75%

    C. 25%

    D. 2%

85. In the guidelines developed by the Child and Adolescent Bipolar Foundation (CABF) for bipolar disorder, the use of clozapine was reserved for patients with which criterion?

    A. Non-response to a mood stabilizer

    B. Non-response to two mood stabilizers

    C. Non-response to a mood stabilizer and an atypical antipsychotic

    D. Non-response to combination treatment with three medications

86. What is one reason pediatric bipolar disorder is diagnosed more frequently in the United States?

    A. Diagnostic differences between DSM and ICD

    B. More thorough diagnostic procedures in the United States

    C. National Association for Mental Illness advocacy

    D. Less strict application of the DSM criteria in youth

87. Which of the following atypical antipsychotics are available in an intramuscular form that can be used emergently?

    A. Olanzapine and ziprasidone

    B. Risperidone and quetiapine

    C. Aripiprazole and quetiapine

    D. Asenapine and olanzapine

88. Venlafaxine has no studies in childhood posttraumatic stress disorder (PTSD) but has strong consensus support in adults. When is the appropriate time to consider its use in children with PTSD?

    A. After two or more failed trials of SSRIs

    B. After a failed tricyclic antidepressant trial

    C. After a failed pimozide trial

    D. After a failed buspirone trial

89. A recent double-blind study of the following antipsychotics in treating 168 children and adolescents with schizophrenia spectrum disorders found no difference in improvement between the groups. Which of the antipsychotics was associated with weight gain and metabolic side effects?

    A. Olanzapine

    B. Molindone

    C. Risperidone

    D. A and C

90. Which of the following is true?

    A. Tics are always involuntary.

    B. Tics can occur during sleep.

    C. Tics represent a displacement of aggressive impulses.

    D. Tics show a caudal–rostral progression.

91. Which of the following medications is the only effective pharmacological approach for giggle incontinence?

    A. Imipramine

    B. DDAVP

    C. Amitriptyline

    D. Methylphenidate

92. Which two neurotransmitters are considered principally involved in attention-deficit/hyperactivity disorder (ADHD)?

    A. Serotonin and dopamine

    B. Glutamate and dopamine

    C. Serotonin and norepinephrine

    D. Norepinephrine and dopamine

    E. None of the above

For questions 93 through 96, match the following types of neurons with the brain structure from which they originate:

93. Cholinergic neurons

94. Dopaminergic neurons

95. Noradrenergic neurons

96. Serotonergic neurons

    A. Raphe nuclei

    B. Substantia nigra and ventral tegmental area

    C. Locus coeruleus

    D. Basal forebrain and brain stem

97. Which statement is TRUE concerning the relative volume of extracellular water in children?

    A. It is high in children and tends to decrease with development.

    B. It is low in children and tends to increase with development.

    C. It is equivalent from childhood through adulthood.

    D. None of the above

98. Which is the most common co-occurring psychiatric disorder in youths with bipolar disorder?

    A. Oppositional defiant disorder

    B. Post-traumatic stress disorder

    C. Major depressive disorder

    D. Attention-deficit/hyperactivity disorder

99. Which of the following led to a decrease in selective serotonin reuptake inhibitor (SSRI) prescriptions near the turn of the 21st century?

    A. Black box warning about suicidal thinking or behaviors

    B. Increased availability of cognitive behavioral therapy

    C. Findings of the Treatment for Adolescents with Depression Study (TADS)

    D. Decrease in public policy initiatives to address depression in youth

100. In addition to improvement in ADHD symptoms, psychostimulants in typically developing children also provide improvement in:

    A. Disruptive behavior

    B. Psychotic symptoms

    C. Obsessive-compulsive symptoms

    D. Stereotypies

101. The main goal during the acute phase of treatment for major depressive disorder (MDD) is to achieve significant clinical response. Approximately how long does this phase last?

    A. 2 weeks

    B. 4 to 6 weeks

    C. 6 to 8 weeks

    D. 12 weeks

102. A child with no prior medication treatment presents with obsessive-compulsive disorder and Tourette's disorder. Therapy has not been adequate to treat the OCD, and the TD is severely impairing. Which of the following would be the most appropriate medication strategy?

    A. SSRI and atomoxetine

    B. SSRI and clonidine

    C. SSRI and risperidone

    D. SSRI and bupropion

103. When were benzodiazepines first available in the United States market?

    A. 1930

    B. 1960

    C. 1975

    D. 1982

104. The American Academy of Child and Adolescent Psychiatry advises that psychotropic medications be used in a safe and clinically appropriate manner and only as part of a comprehensive treatment plan for youths who are incarcerated. Which of the following statements is accurate?

    A. Medication should not be administered without the youth's agreement, unless there is a court order or a psychiatric emergency.

    B. Medication should be used to compensate for staffing issues.

    C. Medications may be warranted as a punitive measure should the child be a danger to others.

    D. Medications may be prescribed without parental consent, since the court serves *in loco parentis* and can provide consent.

105. International data on psychotropic medications dispensed to youths suggest for the most part that which three countries have the highest prevalence of treated mental illness/use of psychotropics?

    A. Great Britain, United States, New Zealand

    B. France, Sweden, Japan

    C. United States, Canada, Australia

    D. United States, Japan, Germany

106. A 9-year-old girl on valproate presents with lethargy, disorientation, and cognitive deficits. Which adverse effect associated with valproate might explain her symptoms?

    A. Hyperammonemia

    B. Lithium toxicity

    C. Hypothyroidism

    D. Thrombocytopenia

    E. Grand mal seizures

107. Child maltreatment is associated with elevated rates of which of the following diagnoses?

    A. Conduct disorder

    B. Post-traumatic stress disorder

    C. Major depression

    D. All of the above

108. Pharmacodynamics can be defined simply as:

    A. What the body does to the drug

    B. What the drug does to the body

    C. Both of the above

    D. None of the above

109. Studies subsequent to the 1976 report from the International Register of Lithium Babies revealed that the risk of congenital defects after *in utero* exposure to lithium is considerably less than previously estimated. What is the current estimated risk for Ebstein's anomaly after first-trimester exposure to lithium?

    A. 5%

    B. 3%

    C. 1.5%

    D. 0.1%

110. What is the highest frequency of EEG activity in the human brain?

    A. Beta

    B. Alpha

    C. Theta

    D. Delta

111. Identify the appropriate definition for either efficacy or effectiveness as commonly used in clinical trial literature.

    A. Efficacy is usually defined as the ability of a treatment to produce clinically meaningful change in usual practice conditions.

    B. Effectiveness is usually defined as the ability of treatment to decrease relevant symptoms compared to controls under ideal circumstances.

    C. Effectiveness is usually defined as the ability of a treatment to produce clinically meaningful change in usual practice conditions.

    D. Efficacy is usually defined as the ability of a target drug to meet the agreed-upon, well-defined symptom cluster.

112. All the following are considered substitution agents for opiate dependence EXCEPT:

    A. Methadone

    B. L-alpha acetylmethadol (LAAM)

    C. Clonidine

    D. Buprenorphine

113. An outpatient psychiatrist suspects neuroleptic malignant syndrome in a patient. Which of the following would be the most appropriate next step?

    A. Begin hydration.

    B. Provide a prescription for dantrolene.

    C. Obtain a CBC and CPK.

    D. Refer to the emergency room.

114. Gabapentin has been shown to be useful as adjunctive treatment in adults for which of the following disorders?

    A. Acute mania

    B. Major depression

    C. Anxiety

    D. Psychosis

115. Formularies that narrowly restrict medication options have an impact on the notion of:

    A. Beneficence

    B. Autonomy

    C. Nonmaleficence

    D. Distributive justice

116. How much time should pass after the discontinuation of fluoxetine before the initiation of a monoamine oxidase inhibitor?

    A. 2 weeks

    B. 5 weeks

    C. 10 weeks

    D. 16 weeks

117. Adverse events in a trial may lead to unblinding of the clinical investigator. What is the best approach to this problem?

    A. Change clinicians periodically.

    B. Re-randomize the subject.

    C. Formulate a placebo that has a side effect profile likely to mimic the active agent.

    D. Assign one clinician to inquire about adverse effects and adjust dose and another to focus on therapeutic outcomes.

118. Which of the following measures can distribute into a continuum with a mean, median, and mode?

    A. Categorical measure

    B. Continuous measure

    C. Dimensional measure

    D. B and C

119. What is the organ of origin for the hormone leptin?

    A. Adipose tissue

    B. Gastrointestinal tract

    C. Hypothalamus

    D. Kidney

120. When identifying target problems for out-of-control behaviors that might be addressed by pharmacotherapy, all of the following would apply EXCEPT:

    A. Frequency of the behavior

    B. Duration of the behavioral episode

    C. The impact on the family

    D. The child's weight

    E. The situations or events associated with the behavior

121. Prior to the publication of DSM-IV, children presenting with symptoms of pervasive worry typically were classified as suffering from which disorder?

    A. Preoccupied attachment

    B. Overanxious disorder (OAD)

    C. Anxious-ambivalent attachment

    D. Generalized anxiety disorder (GAD)

122. Foods such as brussels sprouts, kale, broccoli, and other similar brassica vegetables induce which CYP enzyme?

    A. CYP1A2

    B. CYP2C9

    C. CYP2C19

    D. CYP2D6

123. Which term describes the addition of methyl groups at discrete cytosines in the genome resulting in gene silencing?

    A. Histone acetylation

    B. Triplet repeats

    C. DNA methylation

    D. Translation

124. The Child Adolescent Services Assessment measures the use of mental health services by children 8 to 18 years of age and has been used in clinical trials to determine:

    A. Cost/benefit analysis of treatment

    B. Future service need

    C. Effectiveness of past treatment

    D. The correct diagnosis

125. Some tertiary amine tricyclic antidepressants are metabolized to a secondary amine, such as amitriptyline, which is metabolized to:

    A. Clomipramine

    B. Trimipramine

    C. Nortriptyline

    D. Desipramine

126. FDA approval of a drug means:

    A. There are at least two randomized, double-blind, placebo-controlled trials showing positive effect of a drug.

    B. A drug company can market the drug for the approved disorder only.

    C. Doctors can prescribe the drug for other disorders and uses.

    D. None of the above

    E. A, B, and C

127. Stimulant treatment for attention-deficit/hyperactivity disorder (ADHD) in adolescents with comorbid substance use disorders has been associated with:

    A. No difference in outcomes

    B. Reduced onset of additional psychiatric comorbidities such as major depressive disorder or anxiety disorders

    C. Increased risk of adult substance use

    D. Reduced substance use but increased psychiatric comorbidities

128. Which of the following is the major inhibitory neurotransmitter in the CNS?

    A. Glutamate

    B. Dopamine

    C. Acetylcholine

    D. GABA

129. Which medication was found to be effective in the treatment of selective mutism?

    A. Buspirone

    B. Fluoxetine

    C. Bupropion

    D. Sertraline

130. The prevalence of childhood-onset schizophrenia is less than one in:
    A. 5000
    B. 10,000
    C. 20,000
    D. 30,000

131. The first action by the FDA intended to improve labeling for pediatric use of new medications was the creation of the:
    A. Pediatric Research Equity Act (PREA) of 2003
    B. Pediatric Use subsection under the Precautions section of labeling in 1979
    C. Food and Drug Administration Modernization Act (FDAMA) of 1997
    D. Food and Drug Administration Amendments Act (FDAAA) of 2007
    E. Pediatric Rule of 1998

132. In which country is a large percentage of prescriptions to youths made up of herbal medicines and plant products?
    A. France
    B. United Kingdom
    C. Canada
    D. Taiwan

133. When a hypertensive crisis occurs from combining monoamine oxidase inhibitors (MAOIs) with tyramine-rich foods, which of the following is the best option for emergency treatment?
    A. Alpha blockers
    B. Beta blockers
    C. Lorazepam
    D. Benztropine

134. Obsessive-compulsive disorder commonly presents with comorbid disorders. What is the rate of comorbidity?
    A. 10%
    B. 20%
    C. 35%
    D. >50%

135. A patient presents to your office saying he would like to discuss using a generic alternative to his brand medication to save money. If you do switch, what is the best method?
    A. Slow cross titration of the two medications
    B. Rapid stop and start of each on day one
    C. Stop the first and see if symptoms emerge
    D. All the above might be acceptable
    E. The patient should not switch medications

136. Which of the following is considered the best instrument to use in assessing eating disorders in children aged 8 to 14 years?
    A. Child Eating Disorder Examination
    B. Eating Disorder Examination
    C. Structured Interview for Anorexia and Bulimia Nervosa
    D. Eating Attitudes Test

137. Psychotic symptoms are present in 16% to 60% of children and adolescents with bipolar disorder. Which symptom is the most common?
    A. Paranoid delusions
    B. Visual hallucinations
    C. Auditory hallucinations
    D. Tactile hallucinations

138. Most persons develop a tolerance to the sedative-hypnotic properties of antihistamines within what time frame?
    A. 2 days
    B. 1 week
    C. 3 months
    D. 6 months

139. In the mid 2000s the drug industry accounted for what percentage of the budget of the American Psychiatric Association?
    A. 5%
    B. 10%
    C. 30%
    D. >75%

140. For weight-restored patients with anorexia nervosa, which of the following statements is most accurate?

    A. Weight-restored patients are more likely to relapse while on SSRIs.

    B. Weight-restored patients have a better chance at preventing relapse while on SSRIs.

    C. Weight-restored patients with depression may benefit from SSRIs.

    D. Weight-restored patients are less likely to self-injure while on SSRIs.

141. The current pharmacotherapy of autistic disorder and other pervasive developmental disorders involves targeting all the following symptoms EXCEPT:

    A. The core social impairment of autistic disorder

    B. Irritability and aggression towards others

    C. Interfering repetitive thoughts and behavior

    D. Motor hyperactivity and inattention

    E. Deliberate self-injury

142. Most experts agree that an adequate trial of a serotonin reuptake inhibitor for the treatment of obsessive-compulsive disorder (OCD) should last:

    A. 4 weeks

    B. 8 weeks

    C. 12 weeks

    D. 16 weeks

143. As a rule of thumb, children under which age are less likely to reliably answer questions about mood, time concepts, and comparing themselves to peers and questions that require the child to use judgment?

    A. <6

    B. <9

    C. <12

    D. <15

144. Which of the following amino acids is the immediate precursor for GABA?

    A. Tryptophan

    B. Tyrosine

    C. Serine

    D. Glutamate

145. All of the following are symptoms of serotonin syndrome EXCEPT:

    A. Rigidity

    B. Myoclonus

    C. Hypothermia

    D. Seizures

    E. Delirium

146. What is the purported mechanism of action of antipsychotics in Tourette's disorder?

    A. They decrease dopaminergic input from the substantia nigra into the mesocortex.

    B. They increase dopaminergic input from the prefrontal cortex to the motor cortex.

    C. They decrease dopaminergic input into the tuberoinfundibular region.

    D. They decrease dopaminergic input from the substantia nigra and ventral tegmental area into the basal ganglia.

147. Which best characterizes the elimination of clonidine and guanfacine?

    A. Clonidine is eliminated mostly by liver metabolism.

    B. Guanfacine is eliminated mostly by liver metabolism.

    C. The majority of clonidine is eliminated by renal excretion, while the rest is eliminated by liver metabolism.

    D. Guanfacine is eliminated primarily in the urine.

    E. C and D

148. Several meta-analyses of experimental studies concluded that even moderate doses of alcohol:

    A. Increase the probability of altruistic behaviors

    B. Increase the probability of acting aggressively

    C. Increase the probability of nonproductive behaviors

    D. Increase the probability of morning-after side effects

149. Which of the following agents may be associated with dependence?

    A. Quetiapine

    B. Duloxetine

    C. Pregabalin

    D. Amitriptyline

150. Which governmental act would require manufacturers and other organizations to report on a wide range of payments to physicians and physician-owned entities?

    A. Physician Payments Sunshine Act

    B. Ethics in Government Act

    C. American Recovery and Investment Act

    D. Financial Services Modernization Act

151. Clinical observations in early childhood (36 to 72 months) assessments should include:

    A. Response to minor stressors

    B. Behavioral and affective responses to limit-setting

    C. Themes seen in play

    D. Using caregiver for assistance with regulating behaviors and affect

    E. All of the above

152. Approximately what percentage of patients with attention-deficit/hyperactivity disorder (ADHD) will respond to stimulant treatment if two different stimulant classes are tried consecutively?

    A. 10% to 20%

    B. 25% to 40%

    C. 45% to 60%

    D. 70% to 90%

153. Dietary supplements used by adolescents to enhance sports performance or to lose weight containing which ingredient were banned by the FDA in 2004?

    A. St. John's wort

    B. Gingko biloba

    C. Ephedra

    D. Omega-3 fatty acids

    E. Vitamin D

154. Which of the following is among the most consistent findings in structural MRI studies of mood disorders in adult samples?

    A. Smaller hypothalamic volume

    B. Smaller amygdala volume

    C. Smaller frontal lobe volume

    D. Smaller caudate volume

155. When pediatric autoimmune neuropsychiatric disorder associated with streptococcus (PANDAS) is suspected as an etiology for obsessive-compulsive disorder (OCD), what is the recommended care?

    A. Intravenous immunoglobulin (IVIG)

    B. Plasma exchange

    C. Standard treatments for OCD and streptococcal infection

    D. Antibiotic prophylaxis

156. What is a risk of giving haloperidol intravenously?

    A. Extrapyramidal side effects

    B. Greater QT prolongation and torsades de pointes

    C. Sudden death

    D. All of the above

157. Which of the following approaches has empiric support for the treatment of substance use in adolescents?

    A. Multisystemic therapy

    B. Family therapy

    C. Cognitive behavioral therapy

    D. All of the above

158. Which one of the following classes of psychotropic medications is most often prescribed to preschoolers?

    A. Atypical antipsychotics

    B. Mood stabilizers

    C. Stimulants

    D. Antidepressants

    E. SSRIs

159. Which term describes how well a screening or diagnostic instrument will detect actual disorders and avoid false-negatives?

    A. Reliability

    B. Validity

    C. Sensitivity

    D. Specificity

160. What are phase II trials?

  A. Post-marketing studies to delineate additional information, including the drug's risks, benefits, and optimal use

  B. Initial studies to determine the metabolism and pharmacologic actions of drugs in humans and the side effects associated with increasing doses, and to gain early evidence of effectiveness; may include healthy participants and/or patients

  C. Controlled clinical studies conducted to evaluate the effectiveness of the drug for a particular indication or indications in patients with the disease or condition under study and to determine the common short-term side effects and risks

  D. Expanded controlled and uncontrolled trials after preliminary evidence suggesting effectiveness of the drug has been obtained; intended to gather additional information to evaluate the overall benefit/risk relationship of the drug and provide and adequate basis for physician labeling

161. Which of the following diagnostic instruments for autistic disorder is currently regarded by many as the "gold standard"?

  A. Autism Diagnostic Observation Schedule (ADOS)

  B. Modified Checklist for Autism in Toddlers (M-CHAT)

  C. Autism Diagnostic Interview-Revised (ADI-R)

  D. Social Communication Questionnaire (SCQ)

  E. Ages and Stages Questionnaire (ASQ)

162. Treatment of youths with major depressive disorder (MDD) with fluoxetine is more efficacious than placebo in preventing relapse. What is the peak period for relapse after the initial positive response to treatment?

  A. 4 months

  B. 6 months

  C. 8 months

  D. 1 year

163. What percentage of adolescents hospitalized with bipolar disorder report psychotic symptoms?

  A. 15%

  B. 25%

  C. 50%

  D. 80%

164. Which of the following was developed as a parent or child report to assess broad clinical symptoms of anxiety in children?

  A. Hamilton Anxiety Rating Scale

  B. School Refusal Assessment Questionnaire

  C. Social Phobia and Anxiety Inventory for Children

  D. Multidimensional Anxiety Scale for Children

165. Which of the following is considered a variant of social phobia?

  A. Generalized anxiety disorder

  B. Panic disorder with agoraphobia

  C. Agoraphobia without history of panic disorder

  D. Selective mutism

166. A patient taking carbamazepine develops a serious drug-related rash. Which is the correct option for subsequent treatment?

  A. Continue carbamazepine treatment at a lower dose.

  B. Discontinue carbamazepine treatment and resume after resolution of the rash.

  C. Discontinue carbamazepine treatment.

  D. Continue carbamazepine treatment at the same dose.

167. In what decade did trazodone emerge as a treatment for depression?

  A. 1920s

  B. 1940s

  C. 1960s

  D. 1980s

168. Which of the following is a dietary supplement that has been used throughout Europe since the 1970s for the treatment of a variety of ailments, including depression, osteoarthritis, and liver problems and is a prescription in some countries?

  A. Thioridazine

  B. Calcium

  C. Ginkgo biloba

  D. S-adenosyl methionine

169. For children 18 and under, symptoms of social anxiety disorder must persist for how long before a diagnosis can be made?

    A. 2 months

    B. 3 months

    C. 4 months

    D. 6 months

170. Which is a well-known scale that can be used for systematic screening of mental health in a general medical setting?

    A. Pediatric Symptom Checklist-17

    B. Vanderbilt ADHD Diagnostic Parent Rating Scale

    C. Children's Depression Rating Scale

    D. Diagnostic Interview Schedule for Children

171. What is the number needed to treat (NNT) for fluoxetine in youths with major depressive disorder (MDD)?

    A. 2

    B. 6

    C. 10

    D. 12

172. Bupropion has been studied in the pediatric population for the treatment of what condition?

    A. Major depressive disorder (MDD)

    B. Bulimia nervosa

    C. Attention-deficit/hyperactivity disorder (ADHD)

    D. A and C

173. What is the proper term for genes that may contribute to disease processes?

    A. Dysfunction gene

    B. Initiator gene

    C. Promoter gene

    D. Susceptibility gene

174. An adolescent on the pediatric medical floor presents with an altered mental status and is agitated. The foremost consideration is to:

    A. Start haloperidol.

    B. Determine the medical etiology.

    C. Start a benzodiazepine.

    D. Place in four-point restraints.

175. What is the estimated rate of response to electroconvulsive therapy (ECT) in adults with mania?

    A. 20%

    B. 40%

    C. 60%

    D. 80%

176. Attention-deficit/hyperactivity disorder (ADHD) is:

    A. Highly heritable

    B. Moderately heritable

    C. Poorly heritable

    D. Not heritable

177. If benzodiazepine use is required in the day prior to electroconvulsive therapy (ECT), which of the following medications would be recommended?

    A. Chlordiazepoxide

    B. Diazepam

    C. Oxazepam

    D. Clonazepam

178. Which term describes the probability that a child identified as NOT having the disorder or symptom actually does NOT have it?

    A. Face validity

    B. Content validity

    C. Positive predictive power

    D. Negative predictive power

179. Several studies have demonstrated the efficacy of lithium for children and adolescents with:

    A. Obsessive-compulsive disorder

    B. Tics

    C. Conduct disorder

    D. Attention-deficit/hyperactivity disorder

180. Volumetric magnetic resonance imaging studies and postmortem findings in patients with Tourette's syndrome have found:

    A. Increase in the caudate volume

    B. Decrease in the caudate volume

    C. Increase in the medulla

    D. Decrease in Broca's area

181. What kind of antidepressant mechanism is more prominent in duloxetine and venlafaxine at lower doses?
    A. Serotonergic reuptake inhibition
    B. Noradrenergic reuptake inhibition
    C. Dopamine reuptake inhibition
    D. Glutamate inhibition

182. Which of the following agents is FDA-approved for the treatment of adult bulimia nervosa?
    A. Fluoxetine
    B. Nortriptyline
    C. Sertraline
    D. Mirtazapine
    E. Venlafaxine

183. All of the following tricyclic antidepressants are sedating and have been frequently prescribed for insomnia EXCEPT:
    A. Amitriptyline
    B. Doxepin
    C. Trimipramine
    D. Desipramine

184. Which of the following describes a process of competitive inhibition?
    A. Tight binding to CYP docking site without destroying the site
    B. Reversible binding to CYP docking site
    C. Tight binding to CYP docking site with destruction of the site
    D. High-affinity binding to CYP docking site

185. What is a potential problem of lamotrigine treatment in children with intellectual disability and epilepsy?
    A. There is an increased risk of seizures with treatment.
    B. Visual hallucinations are common.
    C. Parasomnias are common.
    D. Lamotrigine has been shown to lead to behavioral dysregulation.

186. Which of the following antidepressants can be used as adjunctive treatment for insomnia?
    A. Trazodone
    B. Mirtazapine
    C. Venlafaxine
    D. A and B

187. Compared to adults, the rate of clearance of zolpidem in children is:
    A. Half the adult rate
    B. The same as the adult rate
    C. 3 times the adult rate
    D. 10 times the adult rate

188. Which of the following statements is true regarding youths with bipolar disorder in comparison with adults?
    A. Lower rates of cycling
    B. Higher rates of cycling
    C. Fewer distinct episodes
    D. B and C

189. Youth in which of the following ethnic groups are dispensed the most psychotropic medications in the United States?
    A. Black
    B. Hispanic
    C. White
    D. Asian

190. Which of the following is LEAST likely to be a relevant question for a clinical trial?
    A. How does the combination of pharmacotherapy and psychotherapy compare with monotherapy?
    B. What is the motivation for the child and family to enter the trial?
    C. Is it preferable to administer the most intensive (and likely expensive) treatment first, or should this treatment be reserved for patients who have failed less intensive treatments?
    D. In a trial with children and adolescents, do the treatment effects differ among age groups?

191. **What is the mechanism of action of amphet-amines?**

    A. Amphetamine enters vesicles through dopamine and norepinephrine transporters and induces synaptic vesicle depletion of monoamines.

    B. Amphetamine enters vesicles through dopamine transporters and induces synaptic vesicle acquisition of monoamines.

    C. Amphetamine blocks reuptake of vesicles containing monoamines.

    D. Amphetamine induces reuptake of monoamines.

192. **When compared to adults, children on antipsychotics have:**

    A. Higher risk ratios of gaining weight

    B. Lower risk ratios of gaining weight

    C. Equivalent risk ratios of gaining weight

    D. Less appetite stimulation

193. **Due to circadian-mediated alertness in the evening hours prior to sleep, giving sleep medication too early may:**

    A. Induce disinhibited behaviors

    B. Induce dissociative symptoms

    C. Decrease its effectiveness

    D. All of the above

194. **Which term describes the fraction of the drug that reaches the systemic circulation and is available to exert a biological effect on target tissues?**

    A. Distribution

    B. Bioavailability

    C. Administration

    D. Metabolism

195. **Electroconvulsive therapy (ECT) has shown effectiveness in all the following severe psychiatric conditions EXCEPT:**

    A. Psychotic depression

    B. Mania

    C. Catatonia

    D. Autism

196. **Long-term potentiation and long-term depression are neural activities that subserve which cortical function?**

    A. Visual perception

    B. Ocular dominance

    C. Apoptosis

    D. Learning

    E. Neuronal migration

197. **Which phase of drug metabolism involves oxidation, reduction, and hydrolysis?**

    A. Phase I

    B. Phase II

    C. Both

    D. None of the above

198. **What are the main findings of the 14-month phase of the Multimodal Treatment Study for ADHD study (MTA)?**

    A. For the core symptoms of ADHD, behavioral intervention was more effective than medication treatment.

    B. For the core symptoms of ADHD, behavioral intervention and medication treatment were equally effective.

    C. For the core symptoms of ADHD, medication treatment was more effective than behavioral intervention.

    D. For the core symptoms of ADHD, medical or behavioral intervention proved ineffective.

199. **Valerian root has properties similar to which class of medication?**

    A. Antihistamine

    B. Neuroleptic

    C. SSRI

    D. Benzodiazepine

    E. Anticholinergic

200. **Awareness training and competing response training describe which therapeutic modality?**

    A. Cognitive behavioral therapy

    B. Exposure and response prevention

    C. Habit reversal training

    D. Structural therapy

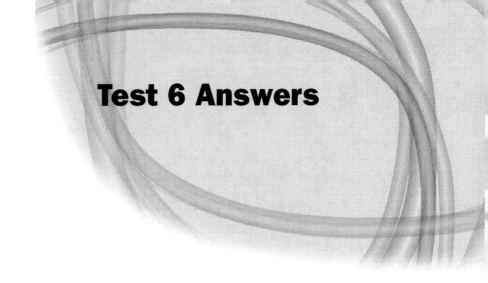

Test 6 Answers

1. Answer: B

Gabapentin modulates calcium influx and influences GABA-ergic transmission. (Chap. 43)

2. Answer: B

Youths with aggression have an annual cost to society six times greater than youths without conduct disturbance. Early aggression (before age 10) presents a poor lifetime prognosis and results in greater hospitalization regardless of diagnosis. (Chap. 47)

3. Answer: A

AACAP suggests baseline assessment of current symptoms, appetite, sleep, height, weight, and cardiovascular status history. (Chap. 18)

4. Answer: C

The specialty of the prescriber is not relevant. The other options would be relevant in helping to guide the appropriateness of psychotropic medication use, although for a given child the question remains complex. (Chap. 49)

5. Answer: D

Internal and external validity are closely related because external validity is specious when lacking good internal validity. (Chap. 29)

6. Answer: C

All the options except group therapy have sufficient evidence to recommend them. Contingency management is another evidence-based option. (Chap. 47)

7. Answer: B

Generally, TAU is treatment in the community as normally delivered. It does not necessarily represent the standard of care, if the care is poorly delivered. (Chap. 50)

8. Answer: E

There a number of modifications to the classic view of basal ganglia function. The answer options include some of those modifications. (Chap. 11)

9. Answer: B

Dopaminergic cells of the ventral tegmental area connect to other brain regions, including the prefrontal cortex, amygdala, hippocampus, and nucleus accumbens. (Chap. 17)

10. Answer: C

No consistent neurohormonal pathophysiology has been identified to explain stimulant-associated height deficits. (Chap. 31)

11. Answer: C

Initial conservative treatment for pediatric nocturnal enuresis involves restricting fluids for 3 hours before bedtime and having the child void at bedtime. (Chap. 48)

12. Answer: E

Gabapentin is structurally similar to GABA. (Chap. 22)

13. Answer: B

The physiological symptomatology may indicate a different neurological substrate for the specific phobia subtype blood/injection/injury. (Chap. 10)

14. Answer: D

The half-life of lamotrigine in children aged 5 to 11 years is 7 hours. (Chap. 22)

15. Answer: C

Ziprasidone and risperidone are likely to have the greatest risk for EPS among the second-generation antipsychotics. (Chap. 37)

16. Answer: A

There have been fewer than 20 articles addressing medication treatment: 8 case reports, 7 open-label studies, 1 chart review, and 3 randomized controlled trials. (Chap. 39)

17. Answer: A

Methylphenidate, D-methylphenidate, and D-amphetamine are short-acting compounds, with onset of action within

30 to 60 minutes and peak effect after 1 to 2 hours, lasting 2 to 5 hours. (Chap. 31)

18. Answer: D

Ramelteon (Rozerem) is a synthetic melatonin receptor agonist that is FDA-approved for the treatment of insomnia. (Chap. 46)

19. Answer: B

The PPWG was established to review existing data regarding the current use of psychotropic medications in preschoolers. The other entities do not exist. (Chap. 51)

20. Answer: C

The traditional agents also include lithium and carbamazepine. (Chap. 22)

21. Answer: B

Deontology posits that the moral aspects of an action are largely irrespective of outcome. (Chap. 52)

22. Answer: A

Since early life stress may contribute to the development of a substance abuse disorder, enriched environment in early life may protect against addiction per animal studies. (Chap. 17)

23. Answer: C

ANC should be monitored weekly for patients on clozapine for the first 6 months, then every 2 weeks for the subsequent 6 months, then monthly. (Chap. 37)

24. Answer: C

The molecule most commonly inserted or uncovered in a phase I reaction is oxygen. Phase I and II reactions are responsible for first-pass effects, in which a substantial fraction of a drug is removed before entering the systemic circulation. (Chap. 4)

25. Answer: A

Hyperglycemia is a concern, not hypoglycemia. The link between antipsychotics and adverse metabolic effects has been well established in adults, but the data in children are more equivocal. (Chap. 23)

26. Answer: C

Dopamine is formed from tyrosine. (Chap. 2)

27. Answer: D

Bupropion is an antidepressant also approved for smoking cessation in adults. (Chap. 41)

28. Answer: B

Dopamine. Norepinephrine is an immediate precursor of epinephrine. (Chap. 2)

29. Answer: D

ICD is more restrictive in its criteria for hyperkinetic disorder (HKD). One study showed that 25% of youths diagnosed with ADHD by DSM-IV would meet the criteria for HKD by ICD-9. (Chap. 54)

30. Answer: A and C

Executive functioning and verbal IQ were inversely associated with physical violence. (Chap. 15)

31. Answer: A

The co-administration of valproic acid and guanfacine can lead to an increase in valproic acid. The exact mechanism is unknown, but both agents are metabolized through glucuronidation, which may lead to competitive inhibition. (Chap. 19)

32. Answer: D

If OCs are discontinued for one week each menstrual cycle, the concentration of lamotrigine increases. It has been recommended that these fluctuations can be avoided by giving OCs throughout the menstrual cycle or by using a progestin-only OC because progestins do not induce glucuronidation. A similar interaction has also been shown to occur with valproic acid and OCs. (Chap. 4)

33. Answer: C

Venlafaxine has a shorter half-life than the others and discontinuation syndrome is more likely; this includes dizziness, headache, body aches, and other flu-like symptoms. (Chap. 21)

34. Answer: D

Somatic symptoms are not a cluster in PTSD. (Chap. 39)

35. Answer: A

Type I error or alpha error is incorrectly rejecting the null hypothesis when the difference is in fact due to chance—that is, saying the treatment made a difference when in fact it did not. (Chap. 50)

36. Answer: D

22q11 deletion syndrome is a risk factor for schizophrenia, autism, and intellectual disability. Cardiac abnormalities can also be present. (Chap. 13)

37. Answer: D

Drug package inserts previously developed are not supported by emerging data. (Chap. 18)

38. Answer: C

IRBs conduct reviews annually. (Chap. 52)

39. Answer: A

Tolerance to sleep improvements on benzodiazepines may occur in 1 to 3 weeks. The other answer options are accurate in their opposites. (Chap. 2)

40. Answer: B

A slow taper for patients on tricyclic antidepressants, dropping the dose by 10 to 25 mg every 2 to 3 days over about 2 weeks, as tolerated, is generally recommended. (Chap. 21)

41. Answer: C

Olanzapine and aripiprazole have relatively minimal effects on QTc. (Chap. 23)

42–46. Answers
42-B, C; 43-C; 44-D; 45-A; 46-B.

These are FDA-labeled indications. Physicians may use medications off-label. (Chap. 51)

47. Answer: C

Sweating, rather than dry skin, is a potential side effect of benzodiazepine withdrawal. Hot and cold flashes, anxiety, depression, feelings of derealization, and perceptual disturbances can also be found. (Chap. 2)

48. Answer: D

Fetal exposure to maternal benzodiazepine use was also associated with an increased risk of NICU admissions and respiratory distress. (Chap. 44)

49. Answer: A

Children less than 6 years old are more prone to develop neurological adverse effects when beginning lithium treatment. (Chap. 22)

50. Answer: B

Routine monitoring of prolactin levels is not recommended for older children prescribed risperidone per new AACAP guidelines in press. (Chap. 45)

51. Answer: A

Sertraline had the lowest and citalopram had the highest umbilical cord to maternal serum concentration. In addition, maternal doses of sertraline and fluoxetine correlated with umbilical cord concentrations, but no such correlation was seen for citalopram or paroxetine (that is, the umbilical cord concentration was independent of the dose the mother was taking). (Chap. 44)

52. Answer: D

An agonist binds to alpha-2 receptors to set this process in motion, not an antagonist. (Chap. 19)

53. Answer: D

An extension of motivational interviewing can also be applied to parents of pediatric patients. (Chap. 30)

54. Answer: C

Most known genetic polymorphisms affect CYP 2D6, increasing the inter-individual variance in antipsychotic levels. (Chap. 23)

55. Answer: D

The optimal valproate level to treat mania in adults is 85 to 110 mg/mL. (Chap. 22)

56. Answer: B

Guanfacine has a longer half-life than clonidine. (Chap. 38)

57. Answer: D

Six-month-old infants of prenatally depressed mothers demonstrate greater negative affect and heightened cortisol response to novel stimuli compared with infants of non-depressed mothers. (Chap. 44)

58. Answer: D

The most common side effect of clonidine is sedation. Hypotension, dry mouth, and confusion are other side effects associated with clonidine. (Chap. 31)

59. Answer: B

Antipsychotics that antagonize D2 are thought to reduce psychosis by their actions in the mesolimbic pathway. Dopamine antagonism in the other brain areas listed leads to unwanted side effects. (Chap. 23)

60. Answer: B

Anorexia is categorized into restricting and binge/purging subgroups. (Chap. 40)

61. Answer: C

Crime statistics indicate that 67% of victims of sexual assault are under age 18; juveniles are the perpetrators for 40% of sexual assault victims less than 6 years old. (Chap. 15)

62. Answer: D

The severity of the ADHD does not seem to make a difference for the effect on aggression. One study found that youths with ADHD respond better to stimulant treatment if they are also aggressive. (Chap. 47)

63. Answer: B

10% to 20% of children who receive psychotropics receive two or more medications. This is not unlike other medical disorders, such as diabetes or HIV, where polypharmacy is the norm, but there is a need for research data and well-designed studies to inform this practice. *(Chap. 49)*

64. Answer: D

Hepatic metabolizing enzymes become saturated even at normal therapeutic concentrations of phenytoin, salicylate, and ethanol. This capacity-limited elimination is best described by zero-order kinetics. (Chap. 3)

65. Answer: A

Sulpiride and tiapride are antipsychotics with weak D2 antagonism. They are not available in the United States but are used for tics and other disorders in Europe. (Chap. 36)

66. Answer: C

The potential side effect of seizures in adults has not been reported in adolescent patients. Headache and scalp pain are the more common side effects of TMS. (Chap. 26)

67. Answer: B

Due to the optimism regarding the selective inhibition of MAO-B on dopamine metabolism and its potential relevance to ADHD, several small trials of selegiline (a selective MAO-B irreversible inhibitor) have been conducted, with mixed results. (Chap. 21)

68. Answer: C

Monoamine oxidase inhibitors (MAOIs) prevent inactivation of biogenic amines. (Chap. 21)

69. Answer: D

The low prevalence, the variable patient population, reluctance to seek help, and at times the medically compromised status of patients make controlled studies difficult. (Chap. 40)

70. Answer: D

The annualized rate of TD in youths in this review was 0.4%, but firm conclusions are precluded by the fact that the studies were not specifically designed to detect TD; also, antipsychotic doses were low and lifetime exposure was relatively short. (Chap. 23)

71. Answer: D

The basal ganglia help create programs to carry out habitual behaviors. (Chap. 11)

72. Answer: B

SSRIs have the best evidence for effectiveness in pediatric anxiety. (Chap. 34)

73. Answer: B

The rate of response to ECT may be more rapid with thrice-weekly sessions, but that frequency may be associated with greater cognitive impairment. (Chap. 26)

74. Answer: A

Alpha agonists have stimulatory effects on growth-hormone secretion through the alpha-2a subtype. (Chap. 19)

75. Answer: A

The prevalence of obsessive-compulsive disorder is 1% to 2%. (Chap. 35)

76. Answer: A

St. John's wort induces the cytochrome P450 system and P-glycoprotein. The effect of OCPs may be decreased with the use of St. John's wort. (Chap. 25)

77. Answer: B

There is evidence that clozapine is superior to other antipsychotics in managing suicidality in adults. (Chap. 37)

78. Answer: B

Gifts, entertainment, and industry-sponsored activities are a form of marketing meant to increase product use by influencing choice and decision-making. (Chap. 53)

79. Answer: D

Stable symptom dimensions in OCD include hoarding, contamination/washing, aggression/checking, and symmetry/ordering. These symptom factors are familial and likely genetic. (Chap. 11)

80. Answer: D

The combination of methylphenidate and clonidine was shown to be superior to either one used alone in the Tourette Syndrome Study Group. This has been found in other trials of ADHD. (Chap. 19)

81. Answer: D

Frequent use of laxatives—about twice weekly—is recommended. Daily high-fiber foods are also recommended. (Chap. 48)

82. Answer: D

The lipid solubility of benzodiazepines means there is an increased accumulation in obese individuals. (Chap. 2)

83. Answer: C

The AMSA PharmFree initiative examines the conflict-of-interest policies of academic medical centers and scores them. (Chap. 53)

84. Answer: D

Only 1% to 2% of the entire body content of serotonin is found in the CNS, as it is found principally in the gut wall and in platelets. (Chap. 2)

85. Answer: D

According to CABF, the use of clozapine in pediatric bipolar disorder is reserved for patients who fail to respond to combination treatment with three medications. (Chap. 33)

86. Answer: D

The diagnostic criteria for DSM and ICD are similar in bipolar disorder. It is the modifying of criteria, or their less strict application, that accounts for pediatric bipolar increases in the United States, among other reasons. (Chap. 54)

87. Answer: A

Olanzapine and ziprasidone are available in IM formulations that can be used in emergencies. Risperidone is available as a depot IM. (Chap. 47)

88. Answer: A

Venlafaxine is a serotonin and norepinephrine reuptake inhibitor and might be considered after a failure of SSRIs. (Chap. 39)

89. Answer: D

This question highlights the recent trend challenging the superiority of second-generation antipsychotics over first-generation antipsychotics. (Chap. 42)

90. Answer: B

Tics can occur during sleep. Tics progress in a rostral–caudal direction. (Chap. 12)

91. Answer: D

Surprisingly, methylphenidate is the only effective pharmacological approach for giggle incontinence, which is the unusual emptying of the bladder in response to severe giggling in urodynamically normal adolescents. (Chap. 48)

92. Answer: D

Norepinephrine and dopamine are the two neurotransmitters principally involved in ADHD. (Chap. 31)

93–96. Answers
93-D; 94-B; 95-C; 96-A. (Chap. 2)

97. Answer: A

Drugs primarily distributed in body water, such as lithium, can have a lower plasma concentration in children compared with adults due to the higher volume of distribution in the pediatric population. (Chap. 3)

98. Answer: D

Bipolar disorder and ADHD are frequently comorbid. Moreover, studies indicate that bipolar disorder is not always an artifact of overlapping criteria between mania and ADHD. (Chap. 33)

99. Answer: A

The black box warning led to a decrease in SSRI prescriptions. (Chap. 49)

100. Answer: A

A review of 14 studies indicated that children with disruptive behavior disorders benefited from stimulant therapy. Effect sizes were moderate to large when reported. (Chap. 42)

101. Answer: D

The two subsequent phases are the continuation and maintenance phases. (Chap. 32)

102. Answer: B

Using an SSRI for the OCD and an alpha agonist for the TD is a reasonable strategy. An antipsychotic might be indicated for severe, debilitating tics, but this is an initial med trial and it would not be one's first choice. (Chap. 35)

103. Answer: B

Chlordiazepoxide, the first available benzodiazepine, was introduced in 1960 and was followed in 1963 by diazepam. (Chap. 2)

104. Answer: A

Medications should not be administered without the youth's assent, unless there is a court order to do so or there is a psychiatric emergency. (Chap. 52)

105. Answer: C

The United States, Canada, and Australia tend to show the highest prevalence. (Chap. 54)

106. Answer: A

Valproate-induced hyperammonemia can be a transient and asymptomatic phenomenon but can become chronic if undetected, and could even lead to coma and death. The risk may increase with the co-administration of other epileptic medications. (Chap. 22)

107. Answer: D

Child maltreatment is also associated with elevated rates of antisocial personality disorder and drug and alcohol problems. (Chap. 8)

108. Answer: B

Pharmacodynamics can be defined as what the drug does to the body. (Chap. 3)

109. Answer: D

The risk of Ebstein's anomaly is 0.1%. Previously, per the International Register of Lithium Babies, the risk for Ebstein's anomaly for newborns exposed to lithium in the first trimester was 2.7%. (Chap. 44)

110. Answer: A

Beta frequencies are 13 to 30 Hz. The predominance of higher frequencies appears to represent greater levels of cortical arousal. (Chap. 15)

111. Answer: C

Effectiveness is usually defined as the ability of a treatment to produce clinically meaningful change in usual practice conditions. Efficacy is usually defined as the ability of treatment to decrease relevant symptoms compared to controls under ideal circumstances. (In this review book, apart from this chapter, the terms are often used interchangeably.) (Chap. 50)

112. Answer: C

Substitution agents in opiate dependence bind to the mu-opiate receptors. Methadone, LAAM, and buprenorphine bind to mu-opiate receptors. (Chap. 41)

113. Answer: D

NMS is an emergency. (Chap. 23)

114. Answer: C

Gabapentin as an adjunct is useful for social phobia and panic disorder in adults. (Chap. 33)

115. Answer: D

Distributive justice refers to the idea that goods and services should be distributed or allocated fairly according to norms, policies, or procedures agreed to by society. (Chap. 52)

116. Answer: B

Fluoxetine has a long half-life and interacts with MAOIs, so at least 5 weeks should elapse before an MAOI is started after fluoxetine discontinuation. (Chap. 20)

117. Answer: D

Placebos may be formulated to provide a side-effect profile similar to the agent being tested, but this has its pitfalls. Another approach is to assign separate investigators to each element of the study. (Chap. 50)

118. Answer: D

Continuous or dimensional measures such as weight or blood pressure would distribute into a continuum of data with a mean, median, and mode. (Chap. 28)

119. Answer: A

The hormone leptin is of crucial significance for the body's adaptation to semi-starvation. (Chap. 16)

120. Answer: D

The child's weight is not relevant to establishing target problems. (Chap. 27)

121. Answer: B

Overanxious disorder (OAD) appeared in the DSM-III and DSM-IIIR, but with the publication of the DSM-IV, this diagnosis was eliminated and children presenting with pervasive worry were diagnosed with GAD. (Chap. 10)

122. Answer: A

CYP1A2 is induced by brassica vegetables. (Chap. 4)

123. Answer: C

DNA methylation is a well-studied epigenetic mechanism that leads to gene silencing by preventing transcription factors and RNA polymerase access to the DNA. (Chap. 8)

124. Answer: A

The CASA assesses services accessed by children and adolescents, from traditional to less formal services, and probes for attitudes and experiences related to treatment; it has been used in clinical trials to help determine costs and benefits of treatment(Chap. 50)

125. Answer: C

Amitriptyline is metabolized to nortriptyline. (Chap. 21)

126. Answer: E

FDA approval has specific implications that are worth knowing. Older drugs may have FDA approval without the current controlled-trial stipulations. (Chap. 20)

127. Answer: B

Stimulant treatment for ADHD in youths with substance use disorders appears to be protective for additional psychiatric disorders. (Chap. 41)

128. Answer: D

GABA is the major inhibitory neurotransmitter in the CNS. Glutamate is the major excitatory neurotransmitter in the CNS. (Chap. 2)

129. Answer: B

Fluoxetine is found helpful in the treatment of selective mutism. (Chap. 42)

130. Answer: D

Childhood-onset schizophrenia is rare and affects less than 1 in 30,000 persons. (Chap. 13)

131. Answer: B

The Pediatric Use subsection includes the standard disclaimer that "safety and effectiveness in children have not been established." In 1994 this Pediatric Use section was updated to allow the FDA to modify pediatric use approval if extrapolation from adult studies and other supporting evidence was sufficient to allow a modification. (Chap. 51)

132. Answer: D

In Taiwan, up to 22% of prescriptions for youths are for herbal medicines or plant products. (Chap. 54)

133. Answer: A

Alpha blockers such as phentolamine are the best option as emergency treatment for a hypertensive crisis. (Chap. 21)

134. Answer: D

Referred and non-referred samples show that the rate of concomitant disorders is well over 50%. These include tics, disruptive behavior disorders, mood disorders, and other anxiety disorders. (Chap. 35)

135. Answer: D

The method of switching medications will depend on drug class, the disease, and the patient in question.

136. Answer: A

The Child Eating Disorder Examination is a modification of the Eating Disorder Examination, developed to be used with children. (Chap. 40)

137. Answer: C

Psychotic symptoms in youths with bipolar disorder may be common, with auditory hallucinations the most common psychotic phenomenon. (Chap. 33)

138. Answer: B

Antihistamines should be used only briefly or as needed for their sedative-hypnotic properties, as tolerance to these effects will develop after 1 week. (Chap. 24)

139. Answer: C

The drug industry accounted for 29% of the APA's budget in 2006. Some 15% was from advertising in APA journals and exhibits at the annual meeting. Another 8% was unrestricted funding for research fellowships and resident conferences, and 6% was from industry-supported symposia at the annual meeting. The APA stated it will phase out the $1.5 million in pharmaceutical company money that it uses to fund continuing medical education. (Chap. 53)

140. Answer: C

SSRIs have not shown much benefit in the treatment of anorexia nervosa. One controlled study found that rates of relapse prevention improve with the use of SSRIs, but this study was seriously biased by a small sample size and a high dropout rate. Another larger study found no benefit. (Chap. 40)

141. Answer: A

Drugs that have a consistent and primary effect on the core social impairment of autism spectrum disorders have not been developed yet. (Chap. 38)

142. Answer: C

Most experts agree than an adequate trial of an SRI should last 10 to 12 weeks at a maximally tolerated dose, even though statistically significant improvement over placebo can be observed by 3 weeks. (Chap. 35)

143. Answer: C

Children less than 12 years of age are less likely to reliably answer questions about mood, time concepts, and comparing themselves to peers and questions that require the child to use judgment. (Chap. 27)

144. Answer: D

GABA is formed after decarboxylation of glutamate by glutamic acid decarboxylase (GAD). (Chap. 2)

145. Answer: C

Hyperthermia rather than hypothermia is a concern in serotonin syndrome. Other signs and symptoms besides those listed are tremors, hyperreflexia, incoordination, autonomic instability, flushing, agitation, seizures, and delirium. (Chap. 20)

146. Answer: D

Antipsychotics, through their D2 receptor antagonism, reduce dopaminergic input into the basal ganglia, thereby reducing tics. (Chap. 36)

147. Answer: E

Elimination of clonidine is 65% by renal excretion and 35% by liver metabolism, while guanfacine and its metabolites are excreted primarily through the urine, with approximately 50% excreted as unchanged drug. (Chap. 19)

148. Answer: B

There is overwhelming evidence that alcohol and aggression are associated; however, the mechanism responsible for the association is unclear. (Chap. 15)

149. Answer: C

Some studies indicate risks for possible dependence on pregabalin treatment. Patients should be monitored for dependence and drug withdrawal upon discontinuation. (Chap. 22)

150.   Answer: A

The Physician Payments Sunshine Act would require yearly reporting of cumulative payments over $100. (Chap. 53)

151.   Answer: E

Observations on how the child uses the caregiver for comfort should also be noted. (Chap. 45)

152.   Answer: D

Of all patients with ADHD, 70% to 90% will respond to stimulant treatment, whether they respond to the first trial or second trial. (Chap. 18)

153.   Answer: C

The FDA banned supplements containing ephedra because of adverse events. (Chap. 25)

154.   Answer: C

MRI and PET studies in adults with mood disorders have reported localized left-sided smaller volume in the subgenual region of the prefrontal cortex. (Chap. 9)

155.   Answer: C

Standard OCD and streptococcal infection care is the standard of care. The other options are experimental. (Chap. 35)

156.   Answer: D

There was an FDA alert in 2007 regarding the revision of labeling for haloperidol use due to its association with torsades de pointes, QT prolongation, and sudden death, especially when given intravenously, even in patients with no preexisting conditions. (Chap. 43)

157.   Answer: D

There is empiric support for MST, family therapy, and CBT for the treatment of adolescent substance use. (Chap. 41)

158.   Answer: C

Stimulants continue to be prescribed to preschoolers more frequently than other psychotropic medications. (Chap. 45)

159.   Answer: C

Sensitivity detects cases while avoiding false-negatives. (Chap. 28)

160.   Answer: C

Phase II trials evaluate the efficacy of the drug in patients with the disease of interest, and help determine the

common short-term adverse events associated with the drug. (Chap. 51)

161.   Answer: C

The ADI-R is a clinician-administered, semi-structured assessment composed of 93 items to aid in the diagnosis of autistic disorder. (Chap. 38)

162.   Answer: A

The peak period of relapse for depressed youths after the initial positive response to fluoxetine treatment is the first 4 months. (Chap. 32)

163.   Answer: D

The majority of children presenting with hallucinations are likely to have an affective disorder and not early-onset schizophrenia spectrum disorder (EOSS). (Chap. 37)

164.   Answer: D

The Screen for Child Anxiety-Related Emotional Disorders (SCARED) is another parent and child report. The other answer options are either clinician-administered (HAM-A) or disorder-specific and not broad measures. (Chap. 34)

165.   Answer: D

Selective mutism is considered a variant of social phobia. (Chap. 34)

166.   Answer: C

Carbamazepine can cause Stevens-Johnson syndrome and toxic epidermal necrolysis and should not be resumed if a patient develops either condition. (Chap. 22)

167.   Answer: D

Trazodone emerged as a treatment for depression in the 1980s. (Chap. 21)

168.   Answer: D

SAMe has randomized controlled trials, mostly European, for adults showing its superiority to placebo for depression. Daily doses in adults are 400 to 1600 mg; in children and adolescents, initial doses of 200 mg have been used. (Chap. 25)

169.   Answer: D

Data from epidemiological studies suggest that social phobia is a common primary diagnosis among adolescents. (Chap. 10)

170.   Answer: A

The Pediatric Symptom Checklist-17 is a screening instrument for a general medical setting. (Chap. 27)

171. Answer: B

The NNT is the number of patients who need to be treated in order to get one response that is attributable to active treatment (and not just to the placebo effect). The NNT for SSRIs in general is 10. It has not been definitively determined why fluoxetine has a better NNT. (Chap. 32)

172. Answer: D

Most of the pediatric clinical trial data for bupropion are for ADHD, and studies indicate superiority over placebo in decreasing ADHD symptoms. One study indicated an effect size roughly half that of stimulants. (Chap. 21)

173. Answer: D

Genes whose mutations increase the predisposition or susceptibility of an individual to develop a disease or disorder are susceptibility genes. (Chap. 6)

174. Answer: B

All the options might be reasonable depending on circumstances, but the foremost consideration is to determine the medical etiology. (Chap. 43)

175. Answer: D

ECT appears to be highly effective for adults with mania. (Chap. 26)

176. Answer: A

ADHD is highly heritable (about .76), which is similar to the heritability of eye color. (Chap. 11)

177. Answer: C

Shorter-acting benzodiazepines are recommended over longer-acting agents, but the medication should not be administered less than 12 hours prior to ECT. (Chap. 26)

178. Answer: D

The negative predictive power describes the test's ability to correctly predict disease-free cases when the test result is negative. (Chap. 28)

179. Answer: C

Several studies have demonstrated the efficacy of lithium for youths with aggression and conduct disorder. (Chap. 22)

180. Answer: B

A decrease in caudate volume has been found in patients with Tourette's syndrome. Studies also suggest cortical thickening and a smaller corpus callosum. (Chap. 12)

181. Answer: A

Duloxetine and venlafaxine are serotonin/norepinephrine reuptake inhibitors; however, at lower doses, both medications have more prominent serotonergic reuptake inhibition. (Chap. 21)

182. Answer: A

In large trials fluoxetine separated from placebo when administered at 60 mg daily; 20 mg was less effective. The tricyclic antidepressants have been found to be effective in reducing binging and purging behaviors but are less often used than SSRIs, given their side-effect profile. (Chap. 40)

183. Answer: D

Desipramine is one of the least sedating tricyclic antidepressants. (Chap. 46)

184. Answer: B

The drug with the higher affinity for the docking site will bind preferentially and "push off" the other drug. Competitive inhibition is less likely to lead to significant interactions than mechanism-based or metabolite-intermediate-complex inhibition. (Chap. 4)

185. Answer: D

Lamotrigine has been shown to lead to behavioral dysregulation in patients with epilepsy and intellectual disability. (Chap. 43)

186. Answer: D

Trazodone should be used with caution in males due to the risk of inducing priapism. (Chap. 32)

187. Answer: C

In adults and children zolpidem reaches peak plasma concentrations 0.75 to 2.6 hours after a dose, and the elimination half-life is 1.5 to 3.2 hours. The rate of clearance in children is 3 times faster than the rate in adults. (Chap. 24)

188. Answer: D

Youths with bipolar disorder have higher rates of cycling with fewer distinct episodes than adults. (Chap. 33)

189. Answer: C

In the United States, fewer African-American, Hispanic, and Asian youths are dispensed psychotropic medications than white youths. (Chap. 53)

190. Answer: B

Motives are least likely to be a relevant question for the trial itself. (Chap. 50)

191. Answer: A

Amphetamine enters vesicles and induces synaptic vesicle depletion. (Chap. 18)

192. Answer: A

Children appear to have higher risk ratios of gaining weight. One olanzapine study, for example, found the risk *ratio for children to be about 4; for adults it was about 3. (Chap. 6)*

193. Answer: D

Circadian-mediated alertness for 1 to 2 hours in the early evening, occurring in both adults and children, can inhibit and complicate the effects of sleep medications. (Chap. 46)

194. Answer: B

The percentage of bioavailability is determined by the total amount absorbed, and the metabolic elimination during first passage through the intestine and liver (first-pass effect for an orally administered drug). (Chap. 3)

195. Answer: D

ECT has been shown effective for psychotic depression, catatonia, and mania in adults. It is not effective for autism. (Chap. 26)

196. Answer: D

Long-term potentiation and depression consist of increases or decreases in synaptic strength that subserve the process of learning. (Chap. 1)

197. Answer: A

Phase I metabolism results in the formation of a more polar compound than the parent molecule. (Chap. 3)

198. Answer: C

The main finding of the 14-month phase of the MTA was that medication treatment was superior to behavioral intervention, and that behavioral intervention did not add to medication effectiveness. (Chap. 31)

199. Answer: D

Valerian has been shown in several studies in adults to have sleep-promoting effects without the "hangover" effects seen with the benzodiazepines, although the effects may not be seen for several weeks. (Chap. 46)

200. Answer: C

Habit reversal training for tic disorders includes awareness training and competing response training. Habit reversal training has been shown to be effective in randomized controlled trials. (Chap. 36)

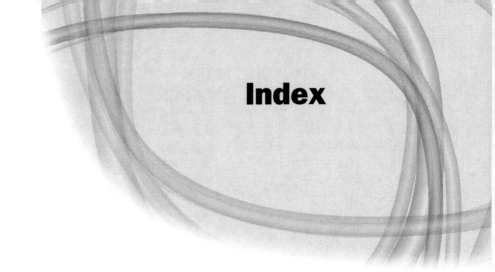

Index

AACAP. *See* American Academy of Child and Adolescent Psychiatry

ABC. *See* Aberrant Behavior Checklist

Aberrant Behavior Checklist (ABC), 70, 85

Abnormal Involuntary Movement Scale (AIMS), 15, 28

absolute neutrophil counts (ANC), 32, 51, 153, 172

absorption, drugs, 6, 23, 39, 55, 63, 76, 82, 88, 101, 103, 116–17, 136, 148

abuse, 5, 23. *See also* child maltreatment; substance abuse
  prevalence of, 99, 115, 136, 148

acamprosate, for substance abuse, 20, 30

acetaldehyde, 139, 149

acetylcholine, 107, 119, 127, 144

active control equivalency study, 16, 28–29

acute dystonia, 70, 85

adaptive skills, 50, 60

ADC. *See* apparent diffusion coefficient

ADHD. *See* attention-deficit/hyperactivity disorder

adipose tissues, 35, 53, 162, 176

ADI-R. *See* Autism Diagnostic Interview-Revised

adolescent substance abuse, 6, 23

adverse events, 16, 29

advertising, 49, 60, 99, 115

aggression, 15, 28. *See also* maladaptive aggression
  alcohol and, 165, 177
  dopamine systems in, 33, 52
  prefrontal cortex and, 76, 88

prevalence of, 136, 148

receptive language deficits and, 34, 53

regulation of, 104, 117

seizures and, 63, 82

treatment for, 1, 4, 9, 21–22, 25, 32, 36, 41, 51, 53, 56, 69, 76, 85, 88, 99, 115, 151, 157, 171, 173

agitation, 48, 59, 139, 149

agranulocytosis, 4, 22

AIMS. *See* Abnormal Involuntary Movement Scale

akathisia, 44, 57, 139, 149

albumin, 48, 59

alcohol, 165, 177
  $GABA_A$ receptor and, 45, 58
  with mirtazapine, 75, 88
  sleep and, 125, 143

alcohol craving, naltrexone for, 12, 26

alcohol dependence, medication for, 20, 30

alcohol intoxication, prefrontal glucose metabolism with, 9, 25

alpha-1 receptor, 108, 119

alpha-2 agonists, 7, 11, 17, 24, 26, 29, 68, 72, 84, 86, 97, 114, 139, 149, 156, 158, 173–74

alpha-2 heteroreceptors, 69, 85

alpha-2 receptors, 7, 24, 36–37, 54, 75, 88, 156, 173

alpha agonists, 139, 149, 161, 175

alpha antagonists, 164, 177

alpha-linolenic acid, 43, 57

alprazolam, 105, 118
  oral contraceptives and, 154, 172

Alzheimer's disease, 64, 82

amantadine, 69, 72, 85, 87

American Academy of Child and Adolescent Psychiatry (AACAP), practice parameters of, 121, 141, 151, 153, 171–72

amitriptyline, 163, 176

amphetamines, 71, 86, 92, 111. *See also* dextroamphetamine
  action of, 153, 170–72, 179
  application of, 93, 112
  mixed salts of, 1, 21

amygdala, 16, 28, 64, 82, 100, 115, 123, 142

amygdalectomy, 99, 115

ANC. *See* absolute neutrophil counts

Angelman, 35, 53

anhedonia, 31, 33, 51–52

anorexia, 157, 173
  treatment for, 49, 60, 105, 118

anorexia nervosa, 64, 83, 165, 177
  depression with, 130, 145
  diagnosis of, 74, 88, 101, 116
  treatment for, 18, 29–30, 37, 54, 75, 88, 129, 145, 158, 174

anterograde amnesia, 5, 23, 96, 113

anticholinergic effects, 40, 56, 66, 83, 129, 144

antidepressants, 32, 51. *See also specific* antidepressants
  for aggression, 32, 51
  application of, 95, 113
  hippocampus neurogenesis and, 1, 21
  REM and, 47, 59
  serotonin syndrome and, 48, 59

antihistamines, 48, 59, 66, 83, 164, 177
  for aggression, 99, 115

Printed in the United States
By Bookmasters